PATHOLOGY FOR RADIOGRAPHERS
AND ALLIED HEALTH PROFESSIONALS

PATHOLOGY FOR RADIOGRAPHERS
and Allied Health Professionals

JOHN A. BLOOMFIELD
M.B., B.S. (London); F.R.A.C.R.; Hon. M.I.R.

Senior Lecturer in Radiology
University of Tasmania
Senior Radiologist
Veterans' Affairs Hospital
Hobart, Australia

YEAR BOOK MEDICAL PUBLISHERS, INC.
Chicago • London

Library of Congress Cataloging in Publication Data

Bloomfield, J. A.
    Pathology for radiographers and allied health
professionals.

    Includes index.
    1. Pathology. 2. Diagnosis, Radioscopic.
3. Radiologic technologists. I. Title. [DNLM:
1. Pathology. 2. Radiography. QZ 4 B655p]
RB112.B58   616.07   81-16501
ISBN 0-8151-0946-6   AACR2

CONTENTS

FOREWORD

PATHOLOGY is the study of disease processes. The role of the diagnostic radiographer is to display *visually* the changes in normal anatomy and tissue density caused by disease. I do not know of any textbook of pathology suitable for radiographers. This work is designed to fill that need.

Although information is given on disease processes in general, I have emphasized those conditions which are of importance to the diagnostic radiographer. This volume, therefore, departs from more formal texts on pathology. Where the nature of the disease process may influence the radiographic technique, attention is drawn to this. I have included a number of uncommon or rare conditions because radiography may play a decisive role in their diagnosis. The functions of the various imaging modalities are indicated where appropriate.

Although my primary aim is to help diagnostic radiographers appreciate the relationship of disease to their specialty, other paramedical groups may find this book of assistance as an introduction to pathology. Understanding disease processes is fundamental knowledge, essential for the healing professions, whose responsibility is the care of the sick.

ACKNOWLEDGMENTS

I WISH TO THANK those people who have contributed in various ways in the preparation of this book. First, I am indebted to those student radiographers who asked me to "recommend a textbook." Finding none suitable for their needs, I was stimulated to undertake this work.

I am grateful to Mr. G. Rowley, Lecturer in Radiography at the Hobart Technical College, and Miss M. Graves, Educational Co-ordinator in the Department of Radiology, University of Virginia Medical Center, for perusing the original draft of the manuscript and encouraging me to proceed with the project.

I am indebted to Mrs. H. Donaldson, Department of Surgery, University of Tasmania, for typing the first draft from my dictaphone tapes. The University of Virginia and, in particular, Dr. T. Keats, Chairman of the Department of Radiology, have been most kind in providing me with facilities to complete the book. I have admired the patience and skill with which Mrs. Pat West and Mrs. Shirley Yowell have produced a coherent script out of the extensively corrected original draft.

Finally, I wish to thank my wife, Jenny, for her encouragement, for her helpful criticisms, and for undertaking the tedious task of proofreading.

GLOSSARY
(Words not defined in the text)

ANAPLASIA. Reversion of cells in a tissue from a highly to a lesser differentiated state.

ATRESIA. Complete blockage of a body tube or orifice due to a congenital cause; e.g., duodenal atresia, pulmonary (valve) atresia.

ATROPHY. Decrease in the size of an organ by loss or shrinkage of its cells; e.g., small kidney from renal artery stenosis.

DIVERTICULUM. Protrusion of the wall of a hollow organ. This may be developmental or acquired. Acquired diverticula usually are of the "pulsion" type; excessive intraluminal pressure forces the mucosa through weakened areas of the organ wall; e.g., pharyngeal pouch. Rarely, adjacent fibrosis distorts the organ wall as it contracts; these are "traction" diverticula; e.g., on midesophagus.

FISTULA. A track connecting two epithelial surfaces; e.g., vesicocolonic fistula connecting urinary bladder and colon.

HYPERPLASIA. Increase in the number of cells in a tissue; e.g., of prostate in men over age 45 years.

HYPERTROPHY.   Increase in the *size* of cells in a tissue; e.g., compensatory in one kidney after loss of the other.

HYPOPLASIA.   Failure of development of an organ or tissue to its full or mature size.

LESION.   A general term to indicate an abnormality in an organ or tissue without specifying its nature.

METAPLASIA.   Repair of a damaged tissue by cells that differ in type from those orginally present; e.g., change in cells of bronchial mucosa following prolonged damage by cigarette smoke.

POLYP.   A growth extending into a cavity from its mucosal surface. It may have a narrow base and be on a stalk (pedunculated) or it may have a broad base (sessile).

SINUS.   A track connecting a deep structure to an epithelial surface; e.g., from infected bone to the skin.

STENOSIS.   A narrowed opening; e.g., mitral (valve) stenosis; or a narrowing of a hollow tube; e.g., hypertrophic pyloric stenosis.

STRICTURE.   A narrowing of a hollow tube, usually fibrous; e.g., esophageal stricture. (This term often is interchangeable with stenosis.)

ULCER.   An area on skin or mucous membrane where the epithelium is missing, with inflammation of the underlying tissue.

1 / BASIC CONCEPTS

"DISEASE is any disturbance of a structure
or of a function of the body, or of any of
its parts."

Symptoms. These are the subjective complaints
that the patient makes when suffering from a disease; e.g., pain, vomiting.

Physical signs. These are the objective findings
that can be observed in the patient suffering from a
disease; e.g., raised temperature, a mass, heart
murmur.

Prognosis. This is a forecast of the likely outcome
of a disease; e.g., a patient with a common cold
will get better in a few days.

Causes of Disease (Etiology)

Often there is more than one cause for a disease
process, especially in elderly patients. However,
causes usually are subdivided into two main
groups.

(1) *Acute;* e.g., germs (bacteria) causing infectious illness.

(2) *Precipitating.* Something that weakens the
normal body defenses and reactions; e.g., leukemia
lowering resistance to infection.

Types of Diseases

INHERITED. Transmitted genetically by the parents; e.g., familial polyposis coli.

CONGENITAL. Present at birth. Some are inherited. Others are acquired during development in utero; e.g., thalidomide poisoning. Most are of unknown cause.

TOXIC. Poisoning by biologic substances; e.g., snakebite; or chemical compounds; e.g., inhaling noxious gases.

INFECTIVE. Invasion by microscopic organisms that multiply within the body, causing harm. Many different organisms can be responsible; e.g., viruses, bacteria, occasionally fungi, helminths (hydatid disease).

TRAUMATIC. Mechanical forces (e.g., direct blow), thermal extremes, electrical currents, or ionizing radiation.

DEGENERATIVE; e.g., aging. Therefore, some diseases occur more in the elderly than in the young; e.g., osteoarthritis.

ALLERGIC. Overreaction of body defenses; e.g., hay fever; reactions to contrast media. (In *autoimmune* diseases, the body overreacts to its own tissues; e.g., rheumatoid arthritis.)

NEOPLASTIC. Cells escape from the processes normally controlling them so that eventually they may destroy the body; e.g., cancer.

NUTRITIONAL. General starvation; failure to obtain a sufficient amount of a specific food item; e.g., rickets due to lack of vitamin D; or secondary to interference with normal digestion and absorption; e.g., celiac disease.

METABOLIC. Derangement of normal physiology; e.g., acromegaly due to excess growth hormone from the pituitary.

IATROGENIC. Caused by medical treatment; e.g., steroid drugs causing collapsed vertebrae; skin cancer after deep x-ray therapy.

Incidence of Disease

MORBIDITY RATE. Morbidity is sickness sufficient to interfere with the normal daily routine of people; e.g., work, recreation. It often is difficult to obtain accurate data on this, and hence to know the true incidence (morbidity rate) of nonfatal diseases in a community.

MORTALITY RATE. This is the number of deaths due to a particular disease, averaged over a population. It indicates the prevalence of that disease in a community.

Death

Somatic Death

This is the decease of the whole body, and occurs when there is permanent failure of the cardiovascular and respiratory systems.

The causes of death tend to be age related. The first month of life is the most dangerous period due to deaths from congenital diseases that cannot be overcome. Five to 14 years has the lowest death rate. The usual cause of death between 15 and 25 years is trauma; e.g., motor car accidents.

In Western communities today, diseases associated with aging predominate because their populations gradually are getting older. Cardiovascular lesions and neoplasia are the most common causes of death. However, it should be noted that infection often is the terminal event in a patient already suffering from another disease.

Cellular Death

The way a cell reacts to an injury will be influenced by the severity and duration of the injury, together with the capacity of the cell to recover. Like the whole body, individual cells also age. The nature of this aging is uncertain but probably is due to the cumulative effects of many mild injuries so that the cell is less and less able to repair itself.

A cell, like the body, dies when it is unable to perform its vital functions, either as a result of severe injury or from aging. Death of a group of cells is termed "necrosis."

Effects of Circulatory Disturbances

These disturbances are commonplace and often have profound effects.

HYPEREMIA. Increased blood in the finer vessels of a tissue. This may be active; e.g., dilatation of arterioles in inflammation; or passive; e.g., obstruction to flow in cardiac failure.

PLETHORA. Overfull vascular tree. This may be seen in the pulmonary vessels in patients with certain forms of congenital heart disease; e.g., left-to-right shunts such as patent atrial septal defect.

OLIGEMIA. Underfilled vascular tree. This may be seen in the pulmonary vessels in patients with certain forms of congenital heart disease; e.g., pulmonary stenosis.

ISCHEMIA. Local decrease or absence of blood supply to an area. This may be sudden; e.g., thrombosis of the femoral artery; or gradual; e.g., renal artery stenosis.

EDEMA. Excess fluid in the cells, the tissues, or the body cavities; e.g., pleural effusion. There are several causes; e.g., lymphatic obstruction by tumor, increased capillary pressure in cardiac failure.

HEMORRHAGE (BLEEDING). Escape of blood from a vessel. This may be due to trauma, disease of the vessel wall, or clotting failure. The effects of a sudden *acute* loss (e.g., cutting a vessel) are very different from those due to a *chronic* slow loss (e.g., bleeding from esophageal varices). Hemorrhage into an organ may destroy it; e.g., a "stroke" is due to bleeding into part of the brain, leading to irreparable damage.

THROMBOSIS. Clot in a vessel forming during life. This may be due to vessel disease; e.g., arteriosclerosis; or to stasis; e.g., deep vein thrombosis.

EMBOLISM. Complete obstruction of a vessel by some object in its lumen. Embolism usually is by a detached thrombus, but tumor cells, air, and other objects can be responsible.

INFARCTION. Death of tissue due to vascular obstruction; e.g., myocardial infarction (heart attack) from blockage of coronary arteries. (*Gangrene* is infarction complicated by infection.)

Inflammation

Inflammation is the local reaction of a tissue to any injurious agent. The agents are many and include physical; e.g., excess irradiation; chemical; e.g., swallowed caustic substance; or living agents; e.g., bacteria. Inflammatory diseases always are given a name ending in "-itis."

Inflammation may be *acute* when the reaction is quick, violent, and lasts hours to days. It is recognized clinically because the lesion is hot, red, swollen, and painful; e.g., a boil due to a staphylococcal infection. Acute inflammations usually give rise to considerable symptoms. *Chronic* inflammations may last weeks to months or even years; e.g., long-standing pulmonary tuberculosis. The patient's symptoms often are milder and less obvious than with an acute infection. There is a whole range of *subacute* inflammations between these extremes.

The outcome of inflammation is variable. For example:

(a) If the damage is mild, healing will be complete; e.g., acute sunburn.

(b) If the damage is severe, cell liquefaction will occur, forming an "abscess." The contents of an abscess are called "pus."

(c) There may be gradual modification of the inflammation, with healing leading to fibrosis. A "granuloma" is a mass or lump of chronic inflammatory tissue.

(d) The agent may not be contained; e.g., general spread of a tuberculous infection (miliary tuberculosis) leading to death of the patient.

Healing (repair) of inflammation occurs in two ways:

(1) Regeneration. New cells arise from pre-existing surviving ones; e.g., liver.

(2) Fibrosis. Where cells cannot regenerate, they are replaced by collagen fibers, forming a "scar"; e.g., in the heart after destruction of its muscle by infarction. Fibrous tissue, as it ages, undergoes contraction, leading to displacement of adjacent structures; e.g., mediastinal shift after lung damage.

Healing is hastened by youth, good nutrition, and local rest of the part. Poor diet, drugs such as steroids, and ionizing radiation all tend to retard it.

Immunity

The immune response is a special defense mechanism by which the body is able to overcome harmful agents; e.g., invading organisms. After the body has been exposed once to the agent (antigen), special lymphocytes (plasma cells) are able to produce rapidly a specific antidote (antibody) to neutralize the noxious agent. This is the basis of immunization programs designed to protect against certain infectious diseases.

Although such a mechanism is of great importance in preventing disease, in some persons, excessive and unnecessary reactions develop to apparently harmless substances; e.g., pollen in hay fever. Such persons are said to be "allergic." If the response is severe enough, the patient develops "anaphylactic shock" and may die from airway obstruction (laryngeal edema) or heart failure unless treated quickly.

Rejection of grafts, e.g., kidney transplant, is due to the immune mechanism destroying the introduced tissue, which it "recognizes" as being foreign. The success of transplant operations is dependent mainly on suppressing the immune reaction to the graft.

The degree of sensitivity of a patient to a particular agent can be tested by injecting a tiny amount of it into the skin and observing the local reaction; e.g., Mantoux test for tuberculosis.

Neoplasia

The radiographer should have a sound understanding of neoplasia to enable her/him to appreciate the key role played by organ imaging in the detection and monitoring of many neoplasms.

The precise meaning of the following terms is important.

NEOPLASM. A focal autonomous growth of tissues with no useful function. It is uncontrolled and not coordinated with other tissues and may be harmful or even fatal to the patient.

TUMOR. Any neoplasm. (Sometimes the term "tumor" is applied to a lump that may not be neoplastic.)

BENIGN TUMOR. A noninvasive neoplasm that remains localized to the area in which it arises.

MALIGNANT TUMOR. A neoplasm with relentless growth, invading the tissues around its margins. It also spreads distantly with lethal effect if not controlled in some way.

CANCER. Any malignant neoplasm. (This term should be differentiated from carcinoma.)

CARCINOGEN. Any agent with a tendency to cause cancer.

CARCINOMA. A malignant neoplasm of epithelium; e.g., bronchogenic carcinoma of the lung.

SARCOMA. A malignant neoplasm of connective tissue; e.g., osteogenic sarcoma of bone.

PRIMARY TUMOR. The malignant neoplasm that occurs first, and from which distant spread eventually occurs.

SECONDARY TUMOR. This refers either to the *contiguous* extension of the primary tumor into adjacent structures or to *distant* spread from the primary site; e.g., carcinoma of the prostate to bones.

METASTATIC TUMOR. A secondary malignant neoplasm that originates from a primary but is separated from it physically.

MULTICENTRIC ORIGIN. A neoplasm arising simultaneously in a number of areas rather than at one site; e.g., lymphoma.

ONCOLOGY. The study of neoplasia.

Benign and malignant tumors differ in many ways and the accompanying table lists the more important differences.

A metastasis is *proof* of malignancy and, with few exceptions, all malignancies metastasize.

Names of Neoplasms

BENIGN. These are named after the tissue, with the suffix "-oma"; e.g., chondroma—benign tumor of cartilage; adenoma—benign tumor of epithelial glands.

MALIGNANT. These are named in various ways: (i) cell of origin; e.g., squamous cell carcinoma; (ii) descriptive; e.g., adenocarcinoma—forming glands; (iii) scirrhous—causing a fibrous reaction; (iv) undifferentiated—lack of identifying tissue pattern.

DIFFERENCES BETWEEN BENIGN AND
MALIGNANT TUMORS

	BENIGN	MALIGNANT
Incidence	Common	Relatively uncommon
Invasiveness	Noninvasive	Invasive
Spread	Localized	Metastatic
Margin	Smooth and encapsulated	Rough, irregular, no capsule
Center	Soft and viable	Firm, unless necrotic
Rate of growth	Slow	Rapid
Microscopy	Resembles normal, with mitoses rare	Often very abnormal with many mitoses

Routes of Metastatic Spread

BLOODSTREAM. Neoplasms may invade walls of veins, with subsequent liberation of masses of tumor cells into the circulation. Emboli from carcinomas of the stomach and colon will circulate through the portal system to lodge in the capillaries of the liver. Carcinomas elsewhere in the body will embolize in the systemic circulation, with arrest of the neoplastic cells in the pulmonary capillaries. Hence, a large proportion of metastases occur in the liver and lungs.

LYMPHATIC SYSTEM. Neoplasms often invade the lymphatic system, giving rise to metastases in two ways. There may be embolization of tumor cells or the malignant cells may grow along lymphatic vessels. Metastases will appear next in the regional lymph nodes, and eventually they may enter the thoracic duct, gaining entry into the bloodstream by this route.

ACROSS SEROSAL CAVITIES. This is uncommon. Carcinoma of the stomach in females may give rise to metastases in the ovaries by transperitoneal seeding.

The distribution and number of metastases depend partly on the length of time the primary has been present and partly on the nature of the primary. Some body tissues, e.g., spleen and skeletal muscle, rarely contain metastases, although the reason for this is obscure.

Causes of Neoplasia

It is not clear in most cases why neoplasia arises. It is probable that more than one mechanism is at work in any individual patient. How the carcinogen acts at the cellular level is also uncertain. It may be due to some failure of the control mechanisms in the cell nucleus. It has been suggested that the body defenses fail to recognize and destroy the abnormal neoplastic cells.

The recognized causes are:

INHERITED. These are rare. Familial polyposis of the colon is a good example. People with this genetic abnormality are born with normal colons but develop innumerable polyps in their colons during adolescence. Malignant changes invariably occur and all these patients die of their colonic carcinomas before they are 45 years old.

IONIZING RADIATION. Either a relatively high dose or exposure over a long time is needed. Many of the early workers with radiation developed squamous cell carcinomas of their hands.

CHEMICAL. The smoke inhaled from cigarettes is the best known example. Other proved carcinogens are asbestos fibers and aniline dyes used in certain industrial processes.

VIRUSES. These are well recognized as causing neoplasms in some animals but none has been proved in man.

Hamartoma. This is a group of lesions in which there is localized disordered development of the tissues; e.g., pulmonary sequestration. Hamartomas present as masses or "tumors" but they are *not* true neoplasms.

Effects of Ionizing Radiation

Excessive ionizing radiation causes cellular damage, although the effects vary with the amount of radiation, the length of time over which it is received, and the cells affected. In general, cells that undergo frequent mitoses, e.g., active red bone marrow and intestinal epithelium, are more susceptible to radiation damage than cells not undergoing mitosis; e.g., adult neurons. A large dose received in a small area will lead to local acute inflammation. A large dose to the whole body will cause widespread changes; e.g., loss of circulating blood corpuscles due to bone marrow damage; diarrhea due to intestinal epithelium damage. If the effects are severe enough, death will ensue in a day or two.

Low doses received over long periods may lead to chronic changes, such as skin atrophy and excessive fibrosis; these may also develop after healing of a local irradiation burn. Repeated low doses may lead to the development of neoplasms; e.g., skin carcinoma, leukemia.

Excessive radiation to the gonads may damage the chromosomes of the ovum or sperm. This increases the mutation rate, so that future generations may have a higher incidence of offspring with congenital defects.

2 / CARDIOVASCULAR SYSTEM

Heart

THE PLAIN CHEST X-RAY is of great value as an aid in the investigation of many heart diseases. If possible, a standard chest film (PA, 2 meters, erect, full inspiration) should be obtained. This often will provide invaluable information about the size and shape of the heart and demonstrate the disturbances of the pulmonary vessels due to the heart lesion.

Congenital Heart Diseases

These are malformations present at birth and often there is more than one. Some are life-threatening and need urgent investigation and treatment. Most of the rest interfere seriously with the heart's function, leading to death before adulthood if not corrected. Many different types occur but those most frequently encountered are listed below.

LEFT-TO-RIGHT SHUNTS. *Atrial septal defect (ASD).* There is a connection between the right and left atria due to a hole in the interatrial septum.

Ventricular septal defect (VSD). There is a connection between the right and left ventricles due to a hole superiorly in the interventricular septum.

Patent ductus arteriosus (PDA). The ductus arteriosus, connecting the distal aortic arch with the left pulmonary artery in the fetus, fails to close after birth.

Anomalous pulmonary venous drainage. One or more pulmonary veins drain into the systemic circulation; e.g., into the inferior vena cava and not the left atrium.

All of these conditions involve passage of blood back into the right side of the heart and the pulmonary circulation, without going around the normal systemic circulation. The lung fields, therefore, are plethoric to a greater or lesser degree. This is seen on the chest x-ray as enlargement of the pulmonary vessels. The heart usually is enlarged due to the increased amount of blood being pumped. Angiocardiography is undertaken to provide accurate detail of the anatomy of the lesion before surgery.

PULMONARY STENOTIC LESIONS. Either the pulmonary artery or the pulmonary valve is narrowed. This reduces the amount of blood reaching the lungs (oligemia), so that the pulmonary vessels on chest x-ray are *smaller* than normal. However, the main pulmonary artery nearly always is *larger* than usual (poststenotic dilatation) due to turbulent flow. The reduced pulmonary blood flow leads to insufficient oxygenation of the blood. These patients, therefore, appear blue (cyanosis); hence, the term "blue babies."

Pulmonary stenosis may be an isolated lesion.

However, in "Fallot's tetralogy," the pulmonary stenosis is combined with a high ventricular septal defect, overriding of the septum by the aorta (thus, it is supplied by both ventricles), and right ventricular hypertrophy (because it has to pump against the pressure of the left ventricle). This condition is investigated by angiocardiography before surgery.

COARCTATION OF THE AORTA. There is marked narrowing or complete blockage of the aorta, usually at the distal end of the aortic arch. To supply sufficient blood to the lower half of the trunk and the lower limbs, many anastomotic vessels develop. These include the intercostal arteries, and the flow in them is reversed so that blood reaches the descending aorta. As they carry a greatly increased volume, they enlarge, become tortuous, and cause pressure erosions of the inferior surfaces of the ribs, giving rise to the well-known sign of "rib notching." The blockage of flow down the aorta raises the blood pressure in the upper limbs and head. This leads to complications; e.g., heart enlargement, cerebral artery aneurysms. A plain chest x-ray will show the rib notching. Prior to surgery, these patients are investigated by aortography to confirm the diagnosis, to demonstrate the size of the narrowing, and to exclude any other congenital cardiac lesions.

TRANSPOSITIONS. In these malformations, the great vessels change position; e.g., the pulmonary artery arises from the left ventricle, the aorta from the right ventricle. Another anomaly connecting the systemic and pulmonary circulations, e.g., septal defect, is necessary to preserve life. Contrast studies are essential to work out the exact anatomy; in particular, a lateral series is needed to identify the reversal of the positions of the pulmonary artery and ascending aorta.

TRUNCUS ARTERIOSUS. In this anomaly, a single vessel arises from both ventricles and supplies branches both to the lungs and to the systemic circulation.

ANOMALIES OF POSITION. The aortic arch may be on the right side though the descending aorta often remains on the left. The heart may be reversed in position (dextrocardia). This may be a solitary anomaly or it may be associated with complete reversal of the position of the liver, intestines, and other abdominal viscera (situs inversus). These anomalies rarely cause any problems to the patient but may confuse the careless radiographer who has not put the left and right markers on correctly!

Acquired Heart Diseases

These are lesions that develop during life due to a variety of etiologic factors.

RHEUMATIC HEART DISEASE. Rheumatic fever is an autoimmune disease in which there are inflammatory changes in many of the connective tissues of the body, usually following a nonspecific infection. The heart valves may be affected and the patient will present months or years after the acute episode with evidence of impaired heart function. The valves affected nearly always are the mitral and aortic because they work at a much higher pressure than those on the right side of the heart. The valve leaflets may be partially fused together, leading to narrowing (stenosis), or they may not close properly, leading to reflux of blood into the atrium during systole (incompetence). Usually there is a mixture of both types of lesions.

The change seen on plain x-ray is enlargement of the heart, with pulmonary vascular congestion, as the blood cannot get through the left side of the heart as readily as through the right side. Calcification may occur in the diseased valves; this may be obvious on plain PA and lateral films or may need tomography for demonstration. The left atrium usually enlarges in both mitral and aortic valvular disease, and this may be demonstrated simply by using a barium swallow. However, for more accurate assessment, angiocardiography with cine studies often is used, as this demonstrates the size of the cardiac chambers, as well as showing the degree of reflux through an incompetent valve or the size of the regurgitant jet through a stenosed valve. Ultrasound (echocardiography) also plays a role in diagnosis, especially in demonstrating the immobility of the mitral valve leaflets.

ISCHEMIC HEART DISEASE. This often is known as coronary heart disease, and is very important clinically. However, since it is basically a disease of the coronary arteries, it is included in the section on Vessels.

CONSTRICTIVE PERICARDITIS. This condition follows inflammatory disease of the pericardium, which becomes fibrosed and eventually may undergo some calcification. Plain chest x-ray will show the calcification, which classically is seen over the right ventricle of the heart and sometimes may extend over the diaphragmatic aspect as well.

CARDIAC FAILURE. Heart failure is present when the heart is unable to pump blood at a rate and volume sufficient to meet normal tissue requirements. Either the right or left ventricle may fail, but often there is a mixture of both.

There are many causes of left ventricular failure. These include hypertension, aortic valve obstruction, and ischemic heart disease. The condition is of some importance to the diagnostic radiographer because many of the changes can be seen on the plain chest film. These include the following.

AN ENLARGED HEART. This may be due to dilatation of its chambers, hypertrophy of its myocardium, a pericardial effusion, or a combination of these.

PULMONARY VASCULAR CONGESTION. Initially there is engorgement of the upper-zone vessels. This is followed by edema, in which the pulmonary alveoli fill up with fluid and therefore lose their normal radiotranslucency. The lungs then are waterlogged and difficult to expand; this often means that a poor inspiratory film is obtained because the patient is unable to breathe in as deeply as usual.

PLEURAL EFFUSIONS. As the heart fails there is accumulation of fluid in all the body cavities.

MISCELLANEOUS. The liver may enlarge and this may be seen on a plain abdominal film. There is physiologic disturbance of other organs such as the kidneys. Patients in cardiac failure should not have IVPs performed, as the renal function is insufficient to provide adequate films.

Vessels

Atheroma

This is the most frequent form of degeneration of the major arteries. It increases in extent and severity as people age, occurring more often in men than in women. It affects vessels such as the aorta, coronary arteries, cerebral arteries, and arteries of the lower limb. Its causes are complex and not entirely understood, but seem to be associated with conditions such as raised blood pressure and increased blood fats (cholesterol).

It is thought that initially cracks occur in the arterial walls. Fatty materials are laid down in the wall deep to these cracks to form raised patches (plaques). These changes are particularly likely to occur where there is movement of the arteries (e.g., proximal coronary arteries) or where there is turbulence of flow (e.g., origin of the internal carotid artery). Later, calcium may be deposited in the atheromatous plaques. If the plaques reach sufficient size, they may obstruct the flow of blood, reducing the amount reaching the capillaries distally, and eventually thrombosis may occur. Occasionally the plaque, which is a weakened area, may rupture.

Plain film radiography usually will not provide information unless the walls of the artery are calcified, when a diagnosis of atheroma can be made. Calcified arterial walls, especially in the iliac and femoral areas, are a very common chance finding when films of these areas are taken in patients over the age of 50 years.

Angiography can be used to make the diagnosis of atheroma and demonstrate its complications, such as occlusion. This often is done when surgery is contemplated in order to allow planning of grafting and bypass procedures.

Coronary Artery Disease

This is the usual etiology of so-called heart attacks. Its main causes seem to be lack of physical exercise, raised blood pressure, raised blood fats, and cigarette smoking. Until recently it was increasing in incidence, but at present there appears to be leveling off and decline in the number of cases.

If the atheroma of the coronary arteries is severe enough, thrombosis will occur so that the muscle distally becomes infarcted. Patients presenting with myocardial infarction often are in shock and seriously ill. Nearly one-quarter of them will die in the first 24 hours, but after that the prognosis improves considerably. Complications include cardiac failure and embolization of clots forming within the cardiac chambers adjacent to the infarcted muscle. In patients who survive extensive infarction, the cardiac muscle is replaced by fibrous tissue. This will restrict movement of the cardiac wall during systole and may even lead to bulging, forming a "ventricular aneurysm." These changes can be shown by angiocardiography and ultrasound.

"Angina pectoris," often called "angina" for short, is the term used to describe attacks of severe pain occurring in the front of the chest, usually after exercise or stress. They are due to reversible ischemia of the heart muscle in patients with atheromatous coronary arteries.

Cineangiography is used to demonstrate the areas of atheroma in the main coronary arteries as an assessment for bypass operations to improve the circulation distally.

Aneurysm

This is "a localized dilatation of an artery." Three main types are recognized.

SACCULAR. There is a localized bulging of the wall like a balloon. A well-known site is the cerebral arteries.

FUSIFORM. There is a circumferential bulging of the wall of the vessel over a considerable distance. This often is seen in the abdominal aortas of elderly people.

DISSECTING. There is a split in the intima, so that the blood passes into the wall separating the inner layers from the adventitia. This usually is seen in the thoracic aorta. An iatrogenic cause is faulty placement of a catheter or needle during angiography, so that the contrast material is injected partly into the wall of the artery and not wholly into the lumen.

The causes of aneurysms are: (i) aging; e.g., dissecting; (ii) infection; e.g., syphilis; (iii) congenital; (iv) trauma—including hypertension.

The term "arteriovenous aneurysm" indicates an abnormal connection between a major artery and vein. This follows trauma and occasionally may complicate needle angiography, especially of the vertebral artery.

Contrast studies are of considerable importance in demonstrating the nature and extent of aneurysms. It should be remembered that sometimes the aneurysm is much larger clinically than is shown by angiography because it may contain a good deal of clot within its lumen. The contrast will outline only that part of the aneurysm that still contains fluid blood.

Hypertension

This means a persistent elevation of the blood pressure. It commonly is taken to refer to the *systemic* circulation. However, *pulmonary* hypertension may occur in chronic lung diseases that narrow the capillary beds. *Portal* hypertension occurs in diseases of the liver where fibrosis obstructs the hepatic capillaries so that there is a rise in pressure in the portal venous system.

In most cases, the cause of systemic hypertension is not known. It becomes more common with advancing age. There is a genetic tendency. Many chronic renal diseases cause hypertension, so radiography plays a part in excluding such conditions; e.g., renal artery stenosis due to atheroma. Endocrine tumors, e.g., pheochromocytoma of the adrenal gland, are a rare cause of hypertension, but radiography is a vital method of demonstrating the site of them.

Venous Thrombosis

Spontaneous thrombosis in the venous system is a common occurrence in hospital patients. Well-recognized causes are:

(a) Stagnation. This is especially likely to occur in patients confined to bed for any length of time, and also in areas where there is local pressure on a part; e.g., the calf when lying in bed.

(b) Recent surgery.

(c) Contraceptive pill.

(d) Neoplasms.

The most common site for venous thrombosis is in the veins of the calf of the leg. In the first few days after thrombosis, the clot lies loosely in the lumen of the vessel. There is the danger that it may become detached and embolize to the lungs, causing pulmonary infarction. If the clot is large, it may completely block the pulmonary arteries, leading to sudden death of the patient. If the clot does not become detached, eventually it will stick to the wall of the vessel and undergo recanalization over a period of some weeks or months.

Radiography plays a vital role in the demonstration of the presence and extent of venous thrombosis, especially in the calf veins. Pulmonary angiography occasionally is used to show the pulmonary emboli.

Phleboliths are small, rounded areas of calcification, developing in old venous thrombi. They are very common in small pelvic veins and are seen in the majority of radiographs of adult lower abdomens. They are of no clinical significance in this area.

3 / RESPIRATORY SYSTEM

RADIOGRAPHY plays a dominant role in the investigation of many problems of the respiratory tract, because the naturally occurring contrast medium, air, allows accurate demonstration of so many of the lesions of the lungs and associated airways. Most respiratory tract diseases are not important as causes of death, except carcinoma of the lung and infection in infants and terminally ill patients.

Upper Respiratory Tract

Congenital Lesions

These are uncommon, but there is one rare condition, "choanal atresia," that is of importance. In this, there is failure of development of the posterior nares so that the nose is not in communication with the nasopharynx. It is an important condition to detect in the newborn, as it interferes with breathing and the ability to suck. It may be demonstrated by instilling contrast material into the nasal cavity with the patient supine.

Infections

SINUSITIS. Infections of the anterior nasal sinuses are a common complication of many common colds. These infections tend to be unilateral, and radiography plays a part in demonstrating their extent. Radiographs will show loss of translucency due to mucosal swelling or, sometimes, to fluid. Erect films will be needed to demonstrate fluid levels if they are present. Radiographically, allergic sinusitis, e.g., hay fever, will give a picture similar to an infectious sinusitis, although usually the allergic sinusitis is bilateral and frequently all the sinuses are involved to a greater or lesser extent. In cases of long-standing allergic sinusitis there may be rounded mucosal swellings visible in the antra due to the formation of polyps.

MASTOIDITIS. Although not paranasal in location, the mastoid air cells also may become infected. As with the anterior nasal sinuses, acute infection may be demonstrated radiographically as a loss of translucency in the air cells. If the infection becomes chronic, the cells are obliterated and the surrounding bone becomes very dense (sclerotic). Resulting debris may form a mass (cholesteatoma), which will erode the surrounding bone.

PHARYNX. Infections of the pharynx are of great importance in the pediatric age group. If the epiglottis is acutely inflamed, it may enlarge rapidly and grossly, so that the child presents in severe respiratory distress; this condition often is a dire emergency. A lateral film of the neck will demonstrate the condition. "Croup" is another inflammatory condition of this region. It is acute laryngotracheitis, with edema of the vocal cords, so once again a lateral film may help in the diagnosis.

Neoplasms

CARCINOMA OF THE PARANASAL SINUSES. This is an uncommon neoplasm. Radiographically, it simulates a sinusitis, but once the carcinoma spreads, it destroys bone. Radiographically, therefore, demonstration of this destruction, often by tomography, is important. Radiography will also show the extent of the soft tissue mass and CT is especially helpful in this regard.

CARCINOMA OF THE LARYNX. This usually takes the form of growths on the vocal cords. Radiography, especially tomography, plays a role in demonstrating the extent of the neoplasm, particularly if it is subglottic in position.

Congenital Lesions

FISSURE ANOMALIES. These are not uncommon, but the only one of any significance to the radiographer is the "azygos lobe." In this, the azygos vein traverses the apical portion of the right lung instead of passing over its hilus. It is readily recognized on a plain chest film but is of no clinical significance.

PULMONARY SEQUESTRATION. In this rare hamartomatous lesion, lung tissue forms without communication with the bronchial tree. It nearly always is left sided. Infection is a frequent complication, so surgical removal of the sequestration is the treatment of choice. Although the mass contains pulmonary structures, its blood supply is from the aorta, often inferior to the diaphragm. An aortogram may be performed prior to operation to demonstrate this blood supply.

Infections

The term "pneumonia" is used to describe infections of the lungs. This usually is an acute condition, and may be a terminal event secondary to the presence of some other disease such as carcinoma.

LOBAR PNEUMONIA. The infection involves one or more lobes and is due to a bacterium, the pneumococcus. It now is an uncommon illness. Patients with lobar pneumonia are acutely ill and many die if not treated. Fortunately, this condition responds readily to antibiotics. The pulmonary alveoli become full of fluid and cells as a result of acute inflammation, and, therefore, on x-ray, the affected lobe appears radiopaque. With appropriate treatment, this resolves, but it should be noted that the clearing of the affected area lags considerably behind the clinical recovery.

BRONCHOPNEUMONIA. There are multiple areas of infection following plugging of the bronchioles by mucus. This often leads to many small abscesses. It nearly always occurs in the basal segments of the lower lobes and usually is bilateral. X-ray will show multiple ill-defined opacities in the lower lobes, often becoming confluent.

ASPIRATION PNEUMONIA. This occurs in patients in whom there is interference with the physiologic mechanisms that prevent inhalation of foreign materials into the airways. It may, therefore, occur in a variety of patients; e.g., during general anesthesia, loss of cough reflex due to old age, or nervous disease. When the contents of the stomach are aspirated there is a rapid onset of a very severe pneumonia, and x-ray will show multiple extensive areas of opacity. Many aspiration pneumonias affect the apical portions of the lower lobes because, in the supine position, the bronchi supplying these areas are the most dependent.

BRONCHIECTASIS. This is a chronic infective process in which extensive destruction of bronchial walls and adjacent lung tissues leads to permanent damage. The bronchi become permanently dilated and contain pus. The dilated bronchi may assume various shapes, such as saccular or cylindrical; hence the names of the various types. This condition used to complicate severe childhood infections; e.g., measles, whooping cough. With the continual decrease in the severity of these conditions, bronchiectasis is being seen less and less frequently. Radiographically, the condition is diagnosed by a bronchogram. This outlines the dilated bronchi and is of importance in demonstrating the extent of the disease prior to surgery.

LUNG ABSCESS. In lung abscess, the infection causes extensive tissue destruction. The destroyed tissues are coughed up, leaving a hole or cavity. If this cavity persists, it develops a thick, fibrous wall and becomes chronic. Lung abscesses follow other conditions such as aspiration pneumonia and neoplasm. On x-ray, they appear as a rounded air space, often with a thickened wall, and may contain fluid, especially if they are in the lower lobe.

HYDATID DISEASE. A hydatid cyst may grow in a lung, which is one of the most common organs affected. As the cyst grows, it will press on a bronchus and eventually rupture into the bronchial tree. X-ray, therefore, will show the various stages of the condition, such as a rounded opacity or an abscess cavity. Calcification of lung hydatids is extremely rare.

FUNGOUS DISEASES. These infections are rare in most parts of the world, although they may occur in patients who are debilitated or on immunosuppressive therapy. Histoplasmosis is endemic in some areas of North America. Usually, the radiographic appearances are not specific. However, in the case of infection with *Aspergillus*, a characteristic appearance may be seen. This fungus affects people who have cavities in their lungs from a previous disease, such as tuberculosis. The fungus grows into a ball in the cavity. This may be seen either on plain films or by tomography, and often moves with changes of position of the patient.

(Tuberculosis is described in the section Pulmonary Fibrosis.)

Asthma

This is a hypersensitivity state. It may be due to noninfective agents; e.g., dusts, pollens. In other cases, it appears that infection plays the dominant role. However, in many patients there is a mixture of these two causes.

The hypersensitivity reaction causes mucosal swelling, production of excess mucus, and bronchiolar muscle spasm. These lead to narrowing of the smaller airways, so that when the patient tries to expire there is trapping of the air in the alveoli. This causes overdistention of the lungs. The radiographer should remember the possibility of overexposing the film, and also of not including the lung bases on the x-ray, because the diaphragm usually is low in position due to its depression by the air trapping. In many patients, the condition is acute, and the hypersensitivity reaction will subside. In others, the condition becomes chronic, so that the air trapping is persistent.

In "status asthmaticus," the patient has severe air trapping, which will not respond to treatment. These patients have severe respiratory difficulties, and the radiographer, when taking a film of such patients, must use the shortest possible exposure time available to get a diagnostic film.

Mechanical Problems

In this section, a group of conditions that cause movement of the structures in the thorax, especially the mediastinum and the diaphragm, are considered. These occur because of volume and pressure changes in the pleural cavity or in the lung itself.

The Pleural Cavity

In the normal person, this is a "potential space." Normally, the visceral and parietal layers of the pleura are in close contact, with a trace of fluid separating them. In various lesions, air and/or fluid may enter this space, so that a wide gap is produced between the chest wall and the underlying lung. Air in the pleural cavity is called a "pneumothorax." Fluid in the pleural cavity is called an "effusion." If both air and fluid occur in the pleural cavity, the condition is referred to as a "hydropneumothorax."

PNEUMOTHORAX. Air may enter the pleural space either from the lung itself or, less frequently, through a hole in the chest wall. A pneumothorax due to a lung lesion may be either "spontaneous," e.g., rupture of a small air cyst (bulla), or caused by some other pulmonary lesion, e.g., abscess near the pleural surface. Air may also enter from a tear of the lung; e.g., fractured rib penetrating the visceral pleura. The most common cause of air entering through the chest wall is, of course, surgery, but it may also follow some forms of trauma; e.g., stab wound.

In a "tension pneumothorax," air continues to enter the pleural space during inspiration but not escape during expiration. This leads to a build-up of pressure in the pleural cavity, which causes movement of structures, especially the mediastinum to the contralateral side. Marked mediastinal shift leads inevitably to various degrees of collapse of the contralateral lung. The diaphragm also becomes depressed and there is a variable widening of the rib spaces.

Radiography plays an important role in the detection and follow-up of pneumothorax. Plain films will show the air in the pleural space, with displacement of the lung away from the chest wall. It can also demonstrate development of a tension pneumothorax.

("Pneumomediastinum" is air in the mediastinum. This condition is seen in a variety of cases; e.g., neonatal respiratory distress and rupture of the esophagus, either spontaneous or after endoscopy. It is included here for completeness.)

PLEURAL EFFUSION. Fluid collects in the pleural space from a number of different causes. This fluid may be a simple "transudate" occurring in conditions such as cardiac failure. If the fluid becomes infected and purulent, the effusion is known as an "empyema." Blood in the pleural space, e.g., after trauma or operation, is known as a "hemothorax."

Rarely, the thoracic duct may become obstructed or divided, leading to the flow of lymph into the pleural space; this is known as a "chylothorax."

The mechanical effects of a pleural effusion are the same as for a pneumothorax, with displacement of the underlying lung, movement of the mediastinum, etc. The degree of these changes depends on the amount of fluid in the pleural space, its rate of accumulation, and the rigidity or otherwise of the mediastinum.

Radiography plays an important role in the demonstration of fluid in the pleural cavity. If the amount of fluid is small, a lateral decubitus film with a horizontal beam often is helpful to demonstrate free fluid running along the lateral chest wall.

The Lung

The volume of the lung in the hemithorax may be either decreased or increased by various conditions. Therefore, changes in mediastinal position and volume of the contralateral lung will occur, similar to those described for pleural lesions.

COLLAPSE (ATELECTASIS). The whole or part of a lung becomes airless and decreased in volume due to bronchial blockage. This may follow:

(a) Lesions in the lumen of the airway; e.g., foreign body.

(b) Lesions growing in the wall; e.g., carcinoma.

(c) Lesions outside the wall, pressing on it; e.g., metastatic nodes.

FIBROSIS. A pre-existing lung disease may cause scarring of the lungs in whole or in part, so that there is diminution in volume due to contraction of this fibrous tissue. This will cause changes in the mediastinal position and in the volumes of any unaffected areas of the lung.

OVERDISTENTION. There is an abnormal increase in volume of a localized area of lung (local emphysema). This follows partial bronchial obstruction; e.g., from a tumor or inhaled foreign body. This causes local air trapping by the same mechanism as described under Asthma.

The total effect of these changes on the rest of the thoracic contents will depend on the extent and rapidity with which they develop. Air trapping will lead to displacements similar to those described for a pneumothorax. Conversely, with the decrease in volume caused by collapse and fibrosis, shifts occur in the reverse direction. These changes cause considerable variation in the radiographic densities, so it may be necessary to adjust exposures or take two films with different techniques to obtain all the diagnostic information required.

Pulmonary Fibrosis

Fibrosis or scarring of the lungs develops from a number of different causes, some of which are discussed below. Depending on the nature of the initial disease, the fibrosis may be either local or generalized. The extent of the fibrosis will influence the severity of the symptoms that the patient may experience.

Tuberculosis

This is an infective disease caused by a bacterium, the acid-fast bacillus (often abbreviated "AFB" on request forms). Most cases are spread by inhalation of infected material from a person already suffering from the disease. The condition is becoming increasingly uncommon in Australia and other Western countries. Patients most at risk today are those with depressed immunity; e.g., immunosuppressive therapy for transplants and cytotoxic treatment for malignancy. Certain occupational groups such as workers in the health field, e.g., radiographers, have an increased chance of contact with infected people and therefore of contracting the condition.

As with other infections there is an initial inflammatory reaction. This may heal, usually with calcification. Sometimes a calcified focus is seen in the periphery of a lobe, with calcification of the lymph nodes at the hilus; this is referred to as a "Ghon's focus." If the infection is not controlled there is extensive, so-called miliary spread of the bacillus, which, if not treated, is rapidly fatal. Occasionally a primary tuberculous infection may present as a pleural effusion with no other radiologic change.

The type of tuberculosis commonly met in clinical practice is the "reinfection phase." There is an alteration in the immune response of the body following the primary infection, which can be shown with a skin test called the "Mantoux test." This results in the secondary infection being a chronic process. Reinfection lesions usually are found in the apices of the lungs, commonly bilateral. Abscess formation with cavitation follows and this often is infective. If this heals, there is fibrosis and, in the latter stages, calcification. Radiography plays an important role in demonstrating the extent of the disease, and especially in the detection of any cavities. Plain films, lordotic views of the apices, and tomography are all important in the radiologic demonstration of tuberculosis.

Sarcoid

This is a disease of unknown cause, and may affect many body systems. However, most cases come to light due to the changes seen on the chest radiograph. In sarcoid, numerous tiny granulomas, a few millimeters across, occur in the organ affected, often with enlargement of the regional lymph nodes. These changes are readily visible on chest x-rays and may be surprisingly extensive in a patient who is clinically well. The multiple small opacities in the lung fields can be mistaken for miliary tuberculosis, but the fact that the patient is not clinically ill rules out the latter diagnosis. In about 80% of cases, the condition clears slowly over some months or a year or two with no long-term effects. Unfortunately, in the remaining 20% of patients, pulmonary fibrosis develops. This usually is apical, and if the previous history is not known, it is easy to confuse with tuberculosis. Such patients have severe respiratory problems.

Pneumoconioses

This is a group of diseases where generalized pulmonary fibrosis follows the inhalation of dust or other particulate matter. Many different substances can cause pneumoconioses, probably the best known being "silicosis."

Silicosis is an intense fibrotic reaction due to inhalation of fine silica particles. Therefore, it is a disease found in people who are miners, grinders, and sandblasters. Such intense fibrotic reaction leads to destruction of much of the functioning lung tissue and therefore to the development of areas of compensatory emphysema. Sometimes large nodular shadows develop in the later stages of the disease, and these may undergo cavitation. The role of radiography in the detection and follow-up of silicosis is obvious.

In recent years, the danger of the inhalation of asbestos fibers has been increasingly recognized. This condition, "asbestosis," is found in people working with the substance. Thus, it may develop in miners and persons manufacturing such items as brake linings and certain insulation materials. The condition causes pleural thickening, and it now is realized that it is carcinogenic. After about 15 years of exposure there is a high incidence of malignancy in both the thorax and abdomen. Of particular interest is the development in many of these patients of a rare pleural tumor—a "mesothelioma."

Radiation Damage

The lungs, like other tissues, will be damaged if irradiated excessively. Such damage is followed by fibrosis, often severe. Radiation fibrosis nearly always follows treatment of malignancies by radiotherapy; e.g., in the lung apex following axillary irradiation for carcinoma of the breast.

Diffuse Interstitial Pulmonary Fibrosis (Hamman-Rich Syndrome)

This may follow a variety of insults to the lungs. It may complicate certain infections or reactions to some drugs, but in many cases the cause is not known. Damaged areas of the lung develop severe fibrosis. Often the distribution of these lesions is irregular and follows no anatomical pattern. Although this condition is rare, radiographers should be aware of its nature. Owing to the severe fibrosis, the ability of the lungs to expand on inspiration is very restricted. Therefore, it may prove very difficult or impossible to obtain satisfactory inspiratory films of these patients.

Emphysema

In this condition, the alveoli distal to the terminal bronchioles become enlarged. This may be due either to overdistention of the alveoli or to the destruction of their walls so that many microscopic spaces become one. The radiographer will realize that in this condition the amount of air becomes increased; thus, it is easy to overexpose the film.

Emphysema may be a generalized disease, although its distribution throughout the lungs may not be uniform. It is probable that the elastic tissue is lost from the interstitium of the lung. Emphysema is common and due to conditions such as repeated infections, obstruction, old age, and heavy cigarette smoking. A chest x-ray will show such changes as a barrel-shaped chest, a decreased transverse cardiac diameter, and a depressed diaphragm, easy to cut off on a PA chest radiograph.

In some cases, the emphysema is "compensatory" in nature. Thus, if a lobe is removed surgically, the adjacent lobe and the contralateral lung will undergo distention to make up for the loss of volume. Sometimes the compensation is generalized in distribution where there is extensive fibrosis.

Fibrocystic Disease (Mucoviscidosis)

This is an inherited disease causing disturbance of function of all the exocrine glands, including the sweat glands. Increased salt secretion in the sweat occurs and this is used to test for the condition.

In the lungs, the bronchial glands may be affected. They then secrete a highly viscous mucus, which is difficult to expel so that there is blocking of the bronchi. This leads to infection. Because of the chronic nature of this condition, it is common for severe bronchiectasis and pulmonary fibrosis to develop.

Neoplasms

Benign Neoplasms

BRONCHIAL ADENOMA. This is an uncommon tumor usually occurring in young adults. Its effects are due to its growth into the bronchial lumen, causing obstruction. Affected patients usually present with recurrent infections and evidence of partial lung collapse. Chest x-rays will show opacity and collapse of the segment of the lung affected. Tomography with or without bronchography may show the tumor, although, more commonly, the diagnosis is made by other means; e.g., bronchoscopy.

Malignant Neoplasms

BRONCHOGENIC CARCINOMA. This is loosely referred to as "lung cancer." It now is the most common primary malignancy in males, and the incidence in females is rising rapidly. Statistics show that the incidence of bronchogenic carcinoma has increased approximately threefold in the past 20 years. Although factors such as atmospheric pollution, asbestosis, and chronic tuberculosis may play a part in the etiology of this lesion, there is no doubt that cigarette smoking is by far the most important cause. Persons who have smoked 40 or more cigarettes a day for 15 years are at great risk of developing this tumor.

Most of the tumors arise in the major bronchi near the lung hili. Many of them are highly anaplastic, the so-called oat cell carcinomas. These often are small and cannot themselves be seen on x-ray. As they grow and encroach on the bronchial lumen, they produce the secondary effects of collapse and recurrent infection. It is these secondary effects rather than the tumor itself that cause most of the opacity on the chest x-ray. As the neoplasm continues to grow and metastasize, mediastinal lymph nodes may enlarge and other complications such as pleural effusions may develop. Ultimately, widespread distant metastases occur, and the prognosis in most cases is extremely poor.

In about 10% of patients, the tumor commences in the more peripheral bronchi and often is symptomless for a long time. A chest x-ray will show a rounded mass in the appropriate part of the lung. Often these patients present only when metastases have occurred, drawing attention to the unsuspected primary.

ALVEOLAR CELL CARCINOMA. This is a rare neoplasm. It usually is multicentric in origin and has a hopeless prognosis. On chest x-ray there are multiple rounded opacities throughout much of the lungs.

PULMONARY METASTASES. Secondary tumors are much more common than primary lung neoplasms. At least 25% of all malignancies develop pulmonary metastases detectable on chest x-ray. Most metastases arise by invasion of a systemic vein and subsequent embolization of tumor cells to the pulmonary capillary bed. Less commonly there may be retrograde lymphatic spread or, rarely, direct invasion by an adjacent tumor. The majority of pulmonary metastases are from carcinomas of the breast, the gastrointestinal tract, the female genital tract, and the kidneys, although any malignant neoplasm may spread in this fashion.

Radiologically there are multiple rounded opacities, often of variable size, throughout the lungs. Occasionally, in a rapidly growing neoplasm, cavitation may occur. There is no means of distinguishing among the various primary sites by observing the nature of opacities seen in the lungs. It is surprising how extensive pulmonary metastases may be and yet the patient has little or no symptomatology connected with the respiratory system. CT scanning is a sensitive method of detecting small metastases before they are visible with conventional radiography.

MESOTHELIOMA. This is a rare neoplasm of the pleura due to pre-existing asbestosis. The tumor causes large soft tissue masses in the pleural cavity, with massive pleural effusions. It has a very poor prognosis.

4 / GASTROINTESTINAL SYSTEM

Congenital Lesions

CONGENITAL LESIONS are present at birth, but some do not present clinically until later in life. Many, however, are life-threatening and demand urgent radiographic investigation before appropriate treatment.

TRACHEOESOPHAGEAL FISTULA. There is atresia of the esophagus at the level of T-4, with the proximal esophagus ending as a blind pouch. In most patients, the distal esophagus is connected by a fistula to the bronchial tree. This condition may be suspected before birth because the inability of the fetus to swallow leads to the development of polyhydramnios (excess amniotic fluid) in the later stages of pregnancy. Radiographic investigation is essential because tracheoesophageal fistula is incompatible with life for more than two or three days. Contrast material is instilled by means of a catheter to demonstrate the blind proximal esophageal pouch. Note that an abdominal x-ray will show gas in the stomach and intestines because of the connection between the bronchial tree and the distal esophageal segment.

DIAPHRAGMATIC HERNIA. During the growth of the diaphragm there may be a failure of certain portions to develop properly, so that communication persists between the thoracic and abdominal cavities. Therefore, various portions of the gut, liver, etc., may be found in the thorax. Radiography plays a role in demonstrating these anatomical abnormalities. It is easy to confuse loops of bowel containing gas with cystic conditions of the lung. However, contrast studies will solve this problem.

HYPERTROPHIC PYLORIC STENOSIS. This condition usually presents in babies around age four to six weeks. There is hypertrophy of the pyloric sphincter so that gastric emptying is delayed, causing vomiting. A barium study may play a role in diagnosis by demonstrating the narrowed, elongated pyloric segment.

SMALL BOWEL ATRESIA. This is most common in the ileum but may occur at any level of the small intestine and often is multiple. The role of radiography is to show, by means of plain films, that an obstruction is present.

MECKEL'S DIVERTICULUM. This is a blind pouch of variable size arising from the distal ileum, due to the persistence of the embryonic yolk sac. It often is symptomless but may cause trouble at any age. Sometimes the small bowel twists around it and becomes obstructed. Alternatively, gastric mucosa may differentiate within the diverticulum and give rise to peptic ulceration, with complications of bleeding and perforation. It often is difficult to visualize the diverticulum radiographically.

MALROTATION. The intestines may not be in the normal position due to failure of the mechanisms of rotation and mesenteric fixation. The most common fault is for the small bowel to be on the right side of the abdomen and the colon on the left. Another type is the persistence of mesenteries for the ascending and descending colons, leading to abnormal mobility. Often these errors of fixation are symptomless, but patients may present at any age with twisting (volvulus) of the bowel. If suspected in the neonatal age group, a barium enema is the quickest and safest method of diagnosis, as it will demonstrate the position of the large bowel.

SITUS INVERSUS. There is a complete reversal of the positions of *all* the abdominal organs, so that the patient is a mirror image of normal. In itself, this is of no consequence to the patient but may cause difficulty in diagnosis if unsuspected. Situs inversus is rare.

DUPLICATION OF THE GUT. This may occur at any level of the gastrointestinal tract. As the name implies, there are two lumens within the gut at a particular level. Usually one of these is blind but occasionally will communicate with the normal lumen. Symptoms are due to enlargement of the obstructed duplication, into which secretion of mucus continues throughout life. Rarely, this pressure is sufficient to cause frank mechanical obstruction.

MECONIUM ILEUS. This is one of the manifestations of mucoviscidosis. It is present in about 10% of cases at birth, due to pancreas involvement. As there is intrauterine failure of secretion of the normal pancreatic enzymes, the meconium in the fetal gut becomes almost solid. Perforation may follow, with the leak of meconium into the peritoneal cavity giving rise to an intense inflammatory reaction. The latter is seen at birth on plain films as an area of calcification. If the perforation does not seal off there will be passage of air into the peritoneal cavity, which can also be detected on x-ray. There also will be evidence of mechanical obstruction of the small bowel.

HIRSCHSPRUNG'S DISEASE. There is absence of neurons in the bowel wall, preventing normal peristalsis. Although this may occur anywhere in the intestines, the vast majority of cases involve the sigmoid colon. The area where the nerve cells are absent fails to relax, so that there is gross dilatation of the bowel proximally. Barium enema shows this narrowing with the proximal dilatation. It is important to remember that these patients should be investigated *without* bowel preparation, as clearing of the impacted feces, by either purgatives or bowel washouts, will remove the evidence of the narrowed segment.

RECTAL ATRESIA. There is failure of development of the distal rectum and anal canal of variable extent. The diagnosis is made readily on clinical inspection. The role of radiography is to demonstrate the distance of the end of the rectum from the skin surface so that surgical repair can be planned. A frequent complication is the presence of a fistula from the rectum to the genitourinary system, commonly the posterior urethra in the male and the vault of the vagina in the female. Both can be demonstrated by contrast studies.

Salivary Glands

CALCULUS. A stone may form in any of the salivary glands and then progress along the duct of the gland. Most stones are calcified and therefore visible on plain films.

INFECTION. Infection may occur, the best known etiology being mumps. If the infection is chronic and repeated there may be destruction of the finer ducts of the gland, giving rise to the condition of "sialectasia," similar to bronchiectasis. This condition may be demonstrated by sialography.

NEOPLASMS. These are uncommon, and most occur in the parotids. The role of radiography is to demonstrate displacement of the ducts by means of sialography.

Esophagus

Pain or difficulty in swallowing is called "dysphagia." This often is well localized by the patient, who will point to the level of the lesion.

CRICOPHARYNGEAL SPASM. The cricopharyngeus muscle is the powerful sphincter that closes the proximal end of the esophagus. This normally relaxes for a brief time to allow the passage of a bolus from the pharynx into the esophagus. In some patients, the opening mechanism becomes disordered so that there is incomplete relaxation. This causes a deep indentation on the posterior wall of the proximal esophagus, seen in the lateral view of a barium swallow.

PHARYNGEAL POUCH. This is a pulsion diverticulum seen in middle-aged and elderly people. It is due to a weakness in the posterior wall of the pharynx at the level of the cricopharyngeus. Once the diverticulum forms there is a tendency for food to go into it rather than down the normal lumen, so that the pouch gets larger and larger. Initially, it remains posterior to the esophagus, but, as it enlarges, it presses on and therefore partially obstructs the esophageal lumen. Eventually, it may present as a mass on the left side of the neck. As it is readily treatable, its recognition by contrast studies is most important.

ESOPHAGEAL WEB. This condition usually is seen in middle-aged women, often with anemia. There is a narrow shelf-like mucosal band lying transversely across the esophagus, causing difficulty in swallowing. Its main importance is that it is premalignant. It can be demonstrated by contrast studies.

ESOPHAGEAL VARICES. These develop in patients with portal hypertension, causing enlargement of the normal communications between the portal and systemic circulations as the blood flow is diverted away from the liver. A common site for this is the distal third of the esophagus, where enlarged, tortuous veins develop, rather like the varicose veins of the leg. Varices may be indirectly demonstrated by a barium study of the esophagus. Alternatively, they may be shown by injecting contrast material into the cardiovascular system, usually by a splenoportogram.

BENIGN STRICTURES. These follow inflammatory lesions. The most common type is a single, usually fairly short, stricture close to the cardia due to reflux esophagitis complicating hiatal hernia. Multiple strictures are much rarer and are due to the swallowing of corrosive substances; e.g., caustic soda, phenol. Contrast studies will demonstrate the site and extent of the strictures.

SPONTANEOUS RUPTURE. This is an unusual condition occurring during violent vomiting. There is splitting of the distal esophagus due to the sudden overdistention, leading to escape of gas and fluid into the mediastinum and left pleural cavity. Plain film radiography is important in demonstrating the pneumomediastinum and left pleural effusion.

CARCINOMA. The most common site for carcinoma is at the level of the tracheal bifurcation, but it may occur in either the upper or lower esophagus. The lesion grows into the lumen of the esophagus, causing narrowing and therefore dysphagia. It also invades adjacent mediastinal structures and may perforate them; e.g., the trachea. Distant metastases are not common in carcinoma of the esophagus.

Cardia

ACHALASIA (CARDIOSPASM). This is a neuromuscular disorder in which there is failure of propagation of normal peristalsis down the esophagus, combined with failure of relaxation of the cardia. This interferes with the passage of food into the stomach, so that the esophagus becomes dilated. The condition is chronic, and patients often do not present for many years after the onset of symptoms. Thus, the esophagus can be of gigantic size when the patient is investigated. In advanced cases there is an esophageal fluid level at the level of the aortic arch due to the retained food. Contrast studies will show the narrowed, elongated segment at the cardia and usually there is no gas bubble in the stomach.

HIATAL HERNIA. As people age, the various orifices in the abdominal wall become weakened and, therefore, the abdominal contents may bulge through into adjacent areas. Hiatal hernia is an example of this; the esophageal opening through the diaphragm becomes lax so that the cardia and adjacent portion of the stomach pass through into the thorax. In the early stages, this is reducible so that the stomach returns back to the abdomen. As time

passes, the defect may become so large that part of
the stomach is permanently located in the thorax.
Associated with the displacement of the cardia into
the thorax there is failure of the normal sphincteric
action so that gastric contents may reflux into the
esophagus, especially when the patient is recum-
bent. This leads to inflammatory changes in the
esophageal mucosa (reflux esophagitis) due to the
action of the gastric juices on it.

Complications may develop as a result of reflux
esophagitis. *Bleeding* may occur from the inflamed
mucosa. If the esophagitis has been severe and
present for a considerable time there may be repair
by fibrosis, leading to a *stricture*. Long-standing reflux esophagitis predisposes to *carcinoma* of the
distal esophagus.

Contrast studies play an important role in the
demonstration of hiatal hernia and its complications.

Stomach

PEPTIC ULCERATION. The mucosa is digested locally
by pepsin in the presence of hydrochloric acid. The
cause of this still is uncertain, but it has been suggested that factors such as nervous tension, irregular meals, and smoking all play a role. It is known
that people who take large doses of aspirin are
prone to develop peptic ulceration. A rare pancreatic tumor also causes peptic ulcerations (Zollinger-Ellison syndrome).

Peptic ulceration often is a chronic disease showing initial healing with later recurrence of the ulceration. Many of the ulcers are located on the lesser curvature. A similar condition is seen in the first part of the duodenum and rarely in a Meckel's diverticulum.

The condition commences as a breach of the mucosa (erosion) due to the digestion by the pepsin. As the condition progresses, the erosion penetrates deeper and deeper into the muscular wall of the stomach, forming an ulcer. Contrast examination will show this ulcer as a protrusion or outpouching of contrast material beyond the apparent lumen of the organ.

Three complications may develop:

(1) *Perforation.* If the erosion penetrates faster than the reparative process in the local stomach wall, it may make a hole through into the peritoneal cavity. Infection of the peritoneal cavity (peritonitis) will ensue, and this is fatal in most cases if not treated. Perforation may be detected with plain films in about 60% of patients by the demonstration of free gas in the peritoneal cavity.

(2) *Bleeding.* Erosion of a vessel by the ulcer may lead to bleeding into the stomach. Altered blood looking like "coffee grounds" may be vomited up (hematemesis). Alternatively, blood may be passed per rectum, making the feces black and tarry (melena). Radiography does not often play a part in the demonstration of gastric bleeding, although selective angiography can show a bleeding artery.

(3) *Obstruction.* This is much less common than the other two. An acute ulcer near the pylorus may

cause obstruction by a mixture of edema and spasm. More proximal ulcers that have been present for a long time may cause obstruction by the formation of a benign stricture, sometimes referred to as an "hourglass" stomach.

NEOPLASMS. Benign tumors of the stomach are uncommon. The most frequent one is a tumor of smooth muscle (leiomyoma).

Carcinoma of the stomach is the most important neoplasm, but its incidence has been declining in Western communities for many years, although it is very common in Japan. Carcinomas may occur anywhere in the stomach, but approximately two-thirds of them are found in the pyloric antrum. Radiography is important in the demonstration of them and three morphologic types are recognized:

(1) *Fungating*. These are masses growing into the lumen of the stomach, and may become large.

(2) *Ulcerating*. These are plaque-like tumors developing ulceration. Some are confused with benign peptic ulcers.

(3) *Infiltrating*. These neoplasms spread within the walls of the stomach, exciting considerable fibrous reaction ("leather bottle" stomach). It is easy to overlook this type on a barium study because often there is rapid passage of contrast material through the stomach. Careful inspection will reveal a small stomach, with rigid walls in the area of the tumor.

Carcinomas spread initially by means of lymphatic infiltration, so metastases occur in the draining lymph nodes. Invasion of the gastric veins leads to metastases in the liver. Hepatic metastases may be shown by CT scanning and ultrasound. More distant spread occurs later in the disease. Prognosis of this condition is poor, and it is doubtful that 10% of patients survive more than five years after diagnosis.

FOREIGN BODIES. Patients swallow an astonishing variety of objects, sometimes accidentally, sometimes by design. Most of these pass from the stomach without trouble. Radiography plays a role in confirming the diagnosis and monitoring the passage of radiopaque foreign bodies from the stomach by means of plain radiography.

A "bezoar" is an accumulation of organic material persisting in the stomach. There are two types. The first is a "phytobezoar," composed of vegetable matter, and most commonly seen in patients after gastric surgery; e.g., vagotomy. The other type is a "trichobezoar," which is a mass of hair, usually found in patients with mental disease.

SURGICAL OPERATIONS. The radiographer should have some knowledge of the various types of operations performed on the stomach. These influence the appearance of the stomach on contrast examination and the rapidity with which the contrast material leaves the organ, or what remains of it. There are five basic operations performed on the stomach:

(1) *Total gastrectomy.* The stomach is completely removed and the esophagus anastomosed to the jejunum. This operation is performed for carcinoma.

(2) *Billroth gastrectomy*. The distal portion of the stomach is removed and the proximal part anastomosed to the first part of the duodenum.

(3) *Polya gastrectomy*. The pyloric antrum is removed and the proximal remnant of the stomach is anastomosed to the proximal jejunum. The proximal end of the duodenum is closed and the duodenal loop is left communicating distally with the jejunum.

(4) *Pyloroplasty with vagotomy*. The vagus nerves are divided at the cardia and the pylorus is refashioned so that it loses its ability to prevent gastric emptying. This is done to control peptic ulceration.

(5) *Gastroenterostomy*. An anastomosis is made between the stomach and the small bowel, usually the jejunum. Gastroenterostomy now is commonly done as a bypass operation should there be some obstructive lesion, such as a neoplasm in the antrum or duodenum. This is a prophylactic measure to spare the patient the misery of persistent and intractable vomiting.

Many gastric operations are complicated sooner or later by abnormal functioning of the small bowel. This leads to varying degrees of malabsorption.

Duodenum

PEPTIC ULCERATION. The first portion of the duodenum, known as the duodenal cap or bulb, is the most common site in the gastrointestinal tract for peptic ulceration. The causes and complications are the same as for the stomach. Duodenal ulcers may occur in any part of the duodenal cap, but the majority develop on the posterior wall. If there has been recurrent ulceration over many years there may be permanent deformity of the cap due to the scarring from the ulceration. Sometimes this causes the cap to resemble a cloverleaf on contrast studies, and it may be referred to as a "trefoil cap."

DIVERTICULUM. Duodenal diverticula, apparently of the acquired pulsion type, are seen with increasing frequency in patients of advancing age. They usually are a chance finding on a contrast examination and rarely give rise to clinical problems.

CARCINOMA. This is rare in the duodenum, especially in the first part.

Intestinal Obstructions

The normal intestines, both small and large, show considerable constant or repeated peristaltic activity as they pass their fluid or semifluid contents distally. Many lesions can interfere with this process, causing obstruction of either the small or large bowel. The obstruction may be *mechanical* or it may be due to a *failure of peristalsis* itself. The causes are as follows:

(1) *Kinking and twisting*. A loop of intestine may kink in an abnormal pocket of the peritoneal cavity; e.g., inguinal hernia. Sometimes a loop with an abnormally long mesentery will undergo twisting; this is known as "volvulus"; e.g., sigmoid volvulus, usually seen in elderly people.

(2) *Narrowing of the lumen.* This may be due to many causes; e.g., foreign body, intussusception, carcinoma, benign stricture, compression by extrinsic mass. The narrowing may be partial or total.

(3) *Failure of peristalsis (paralytic ileus).* Frequently this is seen in patients immediately after abdominal surgery, but may occur in other conditions, such as peritonitis, renal colic, uremia, or following occlusion of a mesenteric vessel.

Once there has been a cessation of flow of the contents of the intestines, the bowel dilates proximally, with accumulation of fluid and/or gas in its lumen. The gas is swallowed whereas the fluid escapes from the intestinal mucosa. The exact effects will depend on the nature of the obstruction. In paralytic ileus, especially in postoperative patients, there tends to be a generalized effect on the whole bowel. When there is a localized lesion in the bowel wall (e.g., stricture, carcinoma), the proximal bowel dilates considerably; at the same time, the bowel distally may be empty, depending on the degree of the obstruction and the length of time it has been present. If a volvulus is complete, it will contain fluid only and will continue to act as an obstructing lesion to the proximal bowel. In sigmoid volvulus, the twisting is incomplete, so that the gas continues to enter the loop, leading to huge distention over the course of a few days.

Where the condition is of sudden onset, it generally is referred to as an "acute abdomen." Plain films, supine and erect, play a very useful role in demonstrating the bowel loops dilated with gas and fluid, which often indicates the level of the obstruction. With more chronic conditions and a slower onset of symptoms there may be a role for contrast studies. An example would be partial obstruction of the colon by carcinoma, diagnosed by contrast enema.

Small Intestine

Diseases of the small bowel, apart from the obstructions, are comparatively rare, and the radiographer is unlikely to see many of them unless working in a specialized gastrointestinal unit.

MALABSORPTION SYNDROME. This is a group of diseases of various causes where there is interference with normal digestion and absorption of small bowel contents. Probably the best known is *celiac disease;* this presents in childhood and is due to sensitivity to the gluten in wheat products, such as bread. The bowel becomes dilated, the mucosal folds atrophied, and there is slowing of peristalsis and even atony. Contrast studies show a dilated bowel with very slow transit times and often "flocculation"; e.g., clumping of barium.

REGIONAL ENTERITIS (CROHN'S DISEASE). This is a chronic inflammatory disease of uncertain cause. It usually presents in young adults and its incidence appears to be increasing. It can affect any part of the gastrointestinal tract but is most common in the small bowel, especially the terminal ileum. In nearly one-fifth of cases, the colon also is involved.

One characteristic of the disease is that it often

affects several levels of the bowel with normal intestine intervening, these being called "skip areas." The lesion starts as mucosal inflammation with ulceration. This excites considerable thickening of the bowel wall. If the disease progresses there is formation of fistulous tracks into the adjacent tissues. The area may also undergo considerable fibrosis, giving rise to mechanical obstruction. Contrast studies often are used to delineate the extent of the disease and to outline possible complications, such as fistulas into the adjacent soft tissues or other organs. If the terminal ileum is severely and chronically involved there may be a long segment of narrowing shown by contrast examination as the "string sign." The disease tends to be self-limiting initially but often relapses, so that patients may be seen repeatedly over many years.

Intussusception

This is an uncommon condition in which there is invagination, like a telescope, of a proximal part of the bowel into its distal part. Two types occur:

(1) *Infantile.* This is seen in young babies, often male. For reasons unknown, the ileum telescopes into the cecum. The mass produced may pass much farther down the colon, and indeed sometimes may present at the anus. If not treated, the part may become gangrenous. Radiography plays a role not only in the diagnosis of the condition but in treatment, as, in many cases, the contrast enema can be used to reduce the intussusception.

(2) *Adult*. The formation of an adult intussusception nearly always is caused by a polyp or some other tumor within the lumen of the bowel. Once again, contrast studies are important in demonstrating the condition, and often its cause.

Neoplasms

These are rare and usually benign.

Appendix

Although inflammation of the appendix (appendicitis) is a common and very important disease, radiography of the appendix is of little value. The appendix, when infected, may undergo perforation, spreading the infection to the peritoneal cavity. Plain abdominal films are of little value in diagnosis of this condition, and usually are taken to exclude other conditions. Where there is chronic infection of the appendix, a calcified stone (fecolith) may develop; this may be identifiable on a plain x-ray film.

Large Intestine

DIVERTICULAR DISEASE. Pulsion diverticula often develop in the colon, and are seen with increasing frequency in patients over the age of 40 years. This condition is called "diverticulosis," and, despite its common occurrence, its cause is obscure. The part of the large bowel most affected is the sigmoid colon. At this level, multiple small diverticula often are found close together along many centimeters of the bowel. Feces may enter these diverticula, become inspissated, causing mucosal erosions, and thus predispose to infection. Inflammation of the diverticula is known as "diverticulitis." This may lead to perforation of the bowel, with abscess formation into the adjacent tissues. Usually, because it is a chronic process, the abscess remains local. Eventually it may rupture into an adjacent organ such as the urinary bladder, forming a permanent connection; e.g., vesicocolic fistula. Patients with such a fistula have persistent urinary tract infections and may notice gas bubbles in their urine during micturition (pneumaturia).

Contrast studies play a vital role in the diagnosis of this condition. The diverticula will be demonstrated in the various parts of the colon, especially the sigmoid. The complications of perforation and fistula formation also can be shown.

NEOPLASMS. *Benign.* Polyps of the large bowel are not uncommon and probably occur in about 10% of the population over the age of 45 years. Many of them are found in the rectal and sigmoid areas. Most of the small ones are benign, but once they exceed 1 cm in diameter, the probability of malignancy becomes much greater. Polyps are shown on contrast studies as rounded lesions, sometimes with an irregular surface and often on a stalk of variable length. Some are mobile and are seen to move during fluoroscopy.

Carcinoma. Carcinoma of the colon is a common lesion and appears to be increasing in frequency. The neoplasm starts as a polypoidal growth of the large bowel wall. As it grows, it spreads around the wall transversely, eventually giving a ring or anular type of lesion, causing narrowing of the whole of the lumen. At least 50% of these carcinomas involve the rectum and sigmoid areas. Occasionally a patient may have more than one carcinoma of the colon, not necessarily arising at the same time. The carcinoma may invade the local tissues. It commonly spreads by lymphatics to the mesenteric nodes and thence to the liver and lungs.

Radiography plays an important role in the demonstration of these lesions. If the carcinoma has grown sufficiently to cause mechanical obstruction, plain films will aid in the diagnosis. In nonobstructive cases, contrast studies are performed to show the level and nature of the lesion.

ULCERATIVE COLITIS. This is an inflammatory lesion of the colonic mucosa. Its cause is not known, although it has been suggested that it is an autoimmune disease. It commonly starts in the rectum, spreads to the sigmoid area, and in severe cases involves the whole of the colon. It tends to be a recurrent condition. In the early stages there is ulceration of the mucosa, with the formation of "pseudopolyps," which are islands of unaffected mucosa. In severe cases, healing proceeds by fibrosis so that there is narrowing and rigidity of sections of the colonic wall. In acute cases there may be paralytic ileus of the colon, with the bowel becoming very dilated (toxic megacolon), and such a colon is likely to perforate. In chronic cases, i.e., colitis present for more than ten years, the risk of a superimposed carcinoma is quite high. Contrast studies are of considerable value in showing the extent of the colitis and in detecting complications.

PNEUMATOSIS COLI. Collections of gas occur in the bowel wall in this uncommon condition. The cause of pneumatosis coli is uncertain, although sometimes it is found in patients with chronic chest disease. It is not due to infection by gas-forming bacteria. Although it may cause nonspecific symptoms, e.g., diarrhea, it is of little significance and resolves spontaneously. It is recognized on contrast enema when areas of gas are seen in the bowel wall.

Liver

HEPATITIS. This is inflammatory disease of the liver cells. It may be due to a variety of causes; e.g., viral infection, toxic chemicals. Some cases apparently are hypersensitivity reactions. The liver has considerable powers of regeneration; thus, in many cases there is complete recovery.

CIRRHOSIS. This is a condition in which there is much fibrous scarring, with nodules of disorganized regenerating liver. Cirrhosis may be the end result of an acute hepatitis or follow other causes; e.g., excessive alcohol abuse and starvation associated with marked lack of protein in the diet. Ultimately, many of these patients develop so much fibrosis that there is interference with the blood flow through the liver, causing portal hypertension and thus the development of portosystemic venous anastomoses; e.g., esophageal varices. Radiography plays little role in the diagnosis of cirrhosis itself but is helpful in elucidating the complication of varices.

The results of long-standing cirrhosis are liver failure and death of the patient. The failure of the hepatic cells causes many serious metabolic changes. Bleeding tendencies develop because the liver is unable to make the clotting factors normally found in blood plasma. This is of importance when patients are investigated by procedures requiring needling; e.g., percutaneous transhepatic cholangiography, splenoportography. Liver failure also causes jaundice.

JAUNDICE (ICTERUS). This is the yellowish discoloration of the skin that appears when there is accumulation of bilirubin in the tissues, and is due to two groups of causes. In the "nonobstructive" group, bilirubin accumulates because the damage to the liver interferes with the excretion of bilirubin. Of more importance to the radiographer is the "obstructive" group, where there is blockage of the biliary system; e.g., by stones, neoplasms, preventing the flow of bile and therefore bilirubin into the duodenum.

SECONDARY NEOPLASMS. These are extremely common, especially from carcinomas occurring in the regions drained by the portal venous system. Apart from demonstrating liver enlargement, which may be huge, plain film radiography has little part in the diagnosis of this condition. However, both ultrasound and CT scanning are able to demonstrate many of the metastatic growths.

PRIMARY CARCINOMA (HEPATOMA). This is an uncommon neoplasm in Western communities. Ultrasound and CT scanning play a role in demonstrating its extent. Many hepatomas are highly vascular and, therefore, may be shown on angiography.

HYDATID DISEASE. The liver is the organ most commonly affected by hydatid disease. Many cysts die after a period of growth, and may be seen many years later as calcified ring-type shadows on plain films. Noncalcified cysts cannot be seen on plain radiography, but both ultrasound and CT scanning can demonstrate them. If the cyst does not die, it will continue to grow and eventually press on and rupture into the biliary tree, giving rise to pain and jaundice.

Gallbladder and Bile Ducts

CONGENITAL LESIONS. A septate gallbladder is seen on oral cholecystography from time to time. In this condition, a transverse mucosal fold or septum divides the gallbladder into two compartments of varying size. If the septum is situated near the fundus of the gallbladder, it sometimes is referred to as a "phrygian gallbladder." Such deformities are of little clinical significance, except that they predispose to the formation of gallstones.

Choledochal cyst is a rare congenital lesion of the common bile duct that undergoes gross cystic dilatation. This usually presents with pain and jaundice in females under the age of ten years. Organ-imaging techniques play a role in diagnosis.

GALLSTONES ("CHOLELITHIASIS"). These are very common, and it is estimated that at least 10% of all persons develop them during the course of their lives. They are more common in females than in males and also are seen more frequently in diabetics, the obese, and in women who have borne children. It is generally agreed that the incidence of gallstones is higher in Australia than anywhere else in the world.

Despite the frequency of gallstones, their formation still is not entirely understood. In some cases, a nidus, e.g., debris after infection, may act as a center on which materials are precipitated out from the bile. However, in the vast majority of cases, substances that normally are in solution in the bile precipitate out for reasons that are obscure but possibly are related to changes in the bile itself. As one of the major roles of the gallbladder is to concentrate bile, it is not surprising that these mechanisms go wrong so frequently.

Gallstones are of variable composition. About

10% of them consist almost entirely of *cholesterol*. These stones often are solitary and may grow to a considerable size, measuring several centimeters across. They do not contain calcium and, therefore, are seen only as filling defects on cholecystography. About the same percentage of stones are of *pure bile pigment*. These are small and dark green and are caused by excess bilirubin excretion from hemolysis (breakdown) of red blood cells. Most gallstones, however, are of *mixed* composition, containing both cholesterol and bile pigment together with a certain amount of calcified material. These stones usually are multiple, faceted, and of different sizes. They will be visible on plain radiography if they contain sufficient calcium, and this occurs in about 10% of stones. Sometimes this calcium is seen on the radiograph as concentric rings, and a similar appearance is seen if the stones are cut; this indicates that they have been formed by a succession of different metabolic processes.

An unknown but considerable number of people go through life with gallstones of which they are unaware, the so-called silent gallstones. However, many stones give rise to symptoms. Once they enter the cystic duct, they cause blockage, which may predispose to infection. If the gallstones are small enough, they may pass into the common bile duct and either impact there or enter the duodenum. Sometimes a gallstone blocked in the gallbladder will ulcerate through its wall into an adjacent organ, usually the duodenum, allowing gas to enter the biliary tree. The stone will pass into the adherent bowel and, if big enough, it may impact, usually in the terminal ileum. This lower small bowel obstruction, associated with a fistula into the gallbladder, is known as "gallstone ileus" and may be diagnosed by means of plain films.

Gallstones can be readily visualized by ultrasound.

CHOLECYSTITIS. This is inflammation of the gallbladder and, although common, its causes are incompletely understood. Infection and obstruction seem to play some part in the development of the condition, but the irritating nature of bile itself undoubtedly is another factor.

Patients with acute cholecystitis often are seriously ill. The prognosis is variable. Some cases subside with few aftereffects. Sometimes gangrene of the wall develops, with rupture of the gallbladder leading to generalized peritonitis. In other cases there is a tendency for the condition to subside, to be followed by recurrent attacks, so that the condition becomes "chronic cholecystitis." Radiology has little role in the diagnosis of this condition, although plain abdominal films may show localized ileus. Ultrasound may provide more useful information by demonstrating an enlarged gallbladder. One rare complication of the condition, "acute pneumocholecystitis," can be diagnosed by radiography, because in this lesion the gallbladder wall contains gas, which is visible on plain films.

As with the acute form, chronic cholecystitis is a disease of little-understood etiology. In addition to the factors mentioned for acute cholecystitis, nearly all patients have gallstones present as well, although it is uncertain whether these are the cause or the effect of the chronic inflammation. Some of these gallbladders will outline on oral cholecystography and then they are seen to be smaller than usual, often with irregularly shaped walls. The gallstones, of course, will also be demonstrated.

CHOLANGITIS. This is infection of the bile ducts. It is a common complication of obstructive lesions.

BENIGN STRICTURES. These may occur in the common bile duct. They commonly follow operations such as cholecystectomy (removal of the gallbladder).

MALIGNANT NEOPLASMS. These are rare in the gallbladder. They may arise anywhere in the biliary tree, but are more common in the distal common bile duct. As the neoplasm grows, it invades the lumen of the biliary tree, leading to pain and eventually jaundice. Percutaneous transhepatic cholangiography is the radiographic technique used to demonstrate the site of such obstructive neoplasms.

Pancreas

PANCREATITIS. This inflammatory lesion of the pancreas may be either acute or chronic. The exact causes of acute pancreatitis are incompletely understood, but basically there is autodigestion of the pancreas due to release of its enzymes into its own tissues. This may be precipitated by factors such as excessive alcohol intake, obstruction of the ampulla of Vater by a gallstone, and contrast injection during duct cannulation. This is a serious condition with a relatively high mortality. If the patient survives, there may be formation of an abscess or of a large fluid collection known as "pseudocyst." Such cysts may reach surprisingly large size, and be shown either on contrast studies by displacement of adjacent organs, e.g., stomach, or, in some patients, more readily by ultrasound or CT scanning.

Chronic pancreatitis is a condition that usually develops after a single acute episode. It is characterized by recurrent attacks of upper abdominal pain; eventually, the pancreas becomes small due to fibrosis and may contain calcified calculi.

NEOPLASMS. Carcinoma is not common. The head of the pancreas is the site of the tumor in about three-quarters of the cases. Diagnosis is not easy by any method and, even at surgery, sometimes it is difficult to distinguish between carcinoma of the head of the pancreas and chronic pancreatitis. As the carcinoma grows, it may cause enlargement of the duodenal loop, which may be demonstrated on barium studies, but this often is a late finding. More recently, the use of ultrasound and CT scanning has enabled the demonstration of masses in the head of the pancreas to be made at an earlier stage. Unfortunately, most patients present when the neoplasm is well advanced and the prognosis is hopeless.

Miscellaneous

ASCITES. This is the accumulation of fluid in the peritoneal cavity. It is due to many causes; e.g., congestive cardiac failure, metastatic malignancy, chronic liver disease. Plain x-ray films play little part in the diagnosis except in advanced cases, where the condition is obvious on clinical grounds anyway. CT scanning has proved to be a much more sensitive method of demonstrating ascites before it can be detected clinically.

PERITONITIS. This is acute inflammation of the peritoneal cavity due to bacterial infection. Most cases follow the perforation of a hollow viscus, e.g., peptic ulcer, and have a fatal outcome if not treated adequately. Radiography plays little or no role in the diagnosis.

Sometimes the infection in the peritoneal cavity is localized to one area. This usually indicates the origin of the abscess; e.g., in the right iliac fossa complicating perforated appendicitis. An abscess localized under the diaphragm is referred to as a "subphrenic abscess." Sometimes it contains organisms producing gas, which can be seen on plain films. This may help in planning surgery, as a plain radiograph showing the presence of gas indicates the site of the abscess.

5 / URINARY SYSTEM

URINARY TRACT DISEASE is recognized clinically by a number of abnormalities. The most common are:

1. *Proteinuria*—the presence of protein in the urine.

2. *Hematuria*—the presence of blood in the urine. This may be obvious on naked-eye inspection of a urine specimen or it may be detectable only by microscopy.

3. *Bacteriuria*—the presence of bacteria in the urine.

4. *Pyuria*—the presence of pus in the urine.

5. *Anuria*—the failure of the kidneys to excrete any urine.

6. *Oliguria*—the formation by the kidneys of very small amounts of urine.

7. *Diuresis*—an increase in the volume of urine excreted by the kidneys.

8. *Renal failure*—this develops when the kidneys are unable to clear the bloodstream of unwanted substances, and may be subdivided into acute and chronic. In *acute* failure there is a sudden cessation of function due to an episode such as shock from trauma or severe burns. This is potentially reversible, although some patients die. In *chronic* failure there is progressive kidney disease extending over

many years before renal function becomes so poor that the patient dies.

9. *Uremia*—the terminal stages of renal failure. These cause widespread changes, such as an increase in the amount of urea in the blood and considerable disturbances of the electrolyte and water balances of the body.

Radiography is extremely important in the diagnosis of many urinary tract diseases. The intravenous pyelogram and other conventional x-ray investigations give invaluable information, but, more recently, CT scanning and ultrasound have provided alternative methods of imaging.

Developmental Defects of the Kidneys

VARIATIONS IN NUMBER OR SIZE. There is a whole range of these lesions, varying from the uncommon "agenesis," where one or both kidneys fail to form, to hypoplastic kidneys and to "duplex" kidneys. In the last there are two pelvicaliceal systems in the kidney, often with separate draining ureters. This condition often, though not invariably, is bilateral.

ABNORMALITIES IN SHAPE AND POSITION. One or the other of the kidneys may be "ectopic" (situated in an abnormal position). This usually takes the form of "malascent" (the kidneys do not reach their normal position in the upper abdomen). This often is associated with other renal tract anomalies. There may be a failure of rotation of the calices so that they may point anteriorly and/or medially instead of laterally. Low-placed kidneys may undergo fusion inferiorly, causing the well-known condition of "horseshoe" kidney. Sometimes the only functioning renal tissue present is in the sacral hollow.

CYSTIC KIDNEYS. The best known of these is "polycystic kidneys," an inherited condition presenting in adults, usually in their thirties. It affects both kidneys, which contain innumerable cysts of various sizes. As life progresses, the cysts enlarge so much that they compress and eventually destroy the normal tissue. Affected patients usually die around the age of 45 years.

Another, much less common, developmental anomaly is "medullary sponge kidney," in which there is dilatation of the collecting tubules. These form cysts in the medulla that often contain numerous small calcified calculi visible on plain films. The cysts will outline with contrast material on IVP. This condition is not always bilateral and may affect only one part of a kidney.

There is a form of cystic disease usually limited to one kidney that occurs in the neonate or infant. It presents as an abdominal mass and is treated by nephrectomy (removal of the kidney).

ARTERIAL ANOMALIES. It is not uncommon for a kidney to have more than one renal artery. Multiple renal arteries are more common in kidneys that are situated more caudally than usual. These extra arteries are important in renal arteriography, as each may have to be catheterized selectively.

URETHRAL VALVES. This is a rare condition of males. Mucosal folds protrude into the posterior urethra, obstructing the flow of urine. The micturating cystourethrogram is a vital method of diagnosis.

Glomerulonephritis

This is an inflammatory reaction caused by hypersensitivity to an infection, usually streptococcal. The antibody produced by the sensitivity interferes with the functioning of the glomeruli. This may be reversible, but in some cases leads to destruction of the glomeruli. Very few patients die in the acute phase, and many recover completely. However, about 20% of patients develop narrowing and scarring of the cortex, leading to chronic renal failure and death.

This condition rarely is investigated by radiography.

Vascular Lesions

The most important of these for the radiographer is "renal artery stenosis," which can be shown by arteriography. Narrowing of the renal artery by atheroma leads to relative ischemia of the kidney, with resultant hypertension. As its blood supply is decreased, the kidney atrophies, and this is recognized on IVP by reduction in its size. Such a kidney often shows an unusually dense delayed pyelogram due to extra water resorption made possible by the slow passage of the glomerular filtrate through the convoluted tubules. If both kidneys are involved there will be increasing renal failure.

Occasionally there is embolization of the renal artery, causing an infarct of the kidney. Thrombosis of the renal vein is of uncertain etiology. It is a cause of the "nephrotic syndrome," which is associated with gross proteinuria.

Infection

PYELONEPHRITIS. This is infection of the calices and renal pelvis. Pyelonephritis may present as an *acute* infection. Any stagnation or obstruction to the passage of urine in any part of the renal tract will predispose to infection. It is not certain how bacteria reach the kidney but it probably is either via the blood supply to the kidneys or by retrograde spread from the urethra, especially in females. Most infections subside with appropriate treatment, and radiography has little role to play in their diagnosis. However, patients who have had more than one urinary tract infection often have an IVP to exclude a treatable cause; e.g., an obstructive lesion.

In *chronic* pyelonephritis, the infection persists so that there is patchy scarring of the kidneys with destruction of many of the calices. This condition complicates "vesicoureteric reflux," in which there is passage of urine from the bladder up the ureter during micturition. The cause appears to be incomplete development of the vesicoureteric junction, as many cases of reflux undergo spontaneous resolution at puberty. If the reflux has been severe and associated with infection there is permanent damage of the kidney, leading to chronic pyelonephritis, eventually complicated by hypertension. Radiography plays an important role in the demonstration of ureteric reflux by means of the micturating cystourethrogram.

TUBERCULOSIS. This now is a rare disease. The infection reaches the kidney via the bloodstream, nearly always from a pre-existing pulmonary lesion. The bacilli lodge in the cortex, causing an abscess. This breaks down, discharging into the caliceal system so that there is a cavity demonstrable by IVP. Healing is shown on the IVP as a cortical scar with associated calcification. If not controlled, the infection spreads down the ureter, which will develop multiple strictures, and thus reaches the bladder. The bladder will become scarred, with considerable reduction in size. Ultimately, if the disease is not treated, infection ascends the other ureter, with involvement of the second kidney.

CYSTITIS. This is inflammation of the bladder, and is much more common in females of all ages than in males. However, it is seen in men, complicating such conditions as obstruction by prostatic hypertrophy or after instrumentation of the bladder; e.g., insertion of a catheter. Radiology plays little part in the diagnosis of cystitis.

RENAL PAPILLARY NECROSIS. The tips of the renal pyramids projecting into the minor calices become infarcted and eventually detached from the rest of the pyramid. Many of these cases are associated with excessive intake of aspirin, but papillary necrosis may complicate other conditions; e.g., diabetes. The condition usually is bilateral, involving several papillae. The IVP is an important diagnostic method, as it will show the absence of the papillae. Often there is considerable destruction of the adjacent pyramid, giving rise to cavities associated with the calices. Although not infective, this lesion is included here for completeness.

Stones

Stones (calculi) occur more frequently in the urinary system than in any other, with the exception of the gallbladder. Most form in the calices or renal pelvis and then pass distally; rarely, they form at other levels such as the bladder. They are found more often in men than in women, especially after the age of 30 years. Infection and obstruction are known predisposing causes.

Urine is a supersaturated solution containing many different crystalline materials, especially calcium and its salts. As with the biliary system, it is easy to appreciate how this situation could be upset so that various substances come out of solution to form particulate matter in the urine. Many factors are known to disturb the normal balance. Concentration of the urine such as may occur in hot weather or in fever is an obvious circumstance where these salts might precipitate out. There may be excessive intake of calcium; e.g., milk diet treatment for peptic ulcer. There may be excessive output of calcium; e.g., decalcification of the skeleton following prolonged bed rest; hyperparathyroidism.

Sometimes people have a metabolic disorder that leads to the excretion of an excessive amount of a particular substance in the urine. An example is gout, where there is abnormal excretion of uric acid. About 5% of urinary tract calculi are uric acid stones. This is important because uric acid stones usually contain little or no calcium and therefore are radiolucent on x-ray. Occasionally there is a "foreign body" in the urinary tract that acts as a nidus for the precipitation of salts from the urine.

Most urinary tract stones are of mixed composition, but nearly half of them contain calcium oxalate with its phosphate and carbonate. They usually are small and, on cutting, show a laminated structure indicating repeated episodes of precipitation.

Renal calculi generally do not give rise to clinical symptoms until they commence to pass from the kidneys. This causes considerable recurrent pain, called "renal colic." This may be associated with other manifestations; e.g., hematuria, frequency of micturition.

Obstructions

The flow of urine through the urinary tract may be obstructed at any level by a variety of lesions. The nature of the obstruction, the level at which it occurs, and the degree of interruption to the flow will influence the effect of the obstruction.

Obstruction may occur in the convoluted tubules due to the deposition of some substance within them; e.g., protein in myelomatosis.

A stone, neoplasm, or disturbance of the neuro-muscular mechanisms can cause obstruction of the pelviureteric junction. The ureter may be obstructed by lesions within it, e.g., stone, neoplasm, or it may be obstructed by extrinsic pressure; e.g., met-astatic nodes, pregnant uterus at the pelvic brim. Obstructions of the bladder usually are due to a stone. Obstructions of the bladder neck are very common in males over the age of 45 due to prostatic hypertrophy. Less frequently, obstructions at this level are due to neurogenic disorders; e.g., paraple-gia from trauma.

Obstructions of the urethra are uncommon, but urethral strictures are seen from time to time in the male, rarely in the female. There are three main causes of stricture formation in the male urethra. These are:

(1) Postinfective; e.g., gonococcal. These stric-tures often are multiple.

(2) Perineal trauma. The membranous urethra tears; healing leaves a single, tight stricture.

(3) Postoperative; e.g., transurethral resection of prostate.

All of these lesions can be shown by retrograde urethrography.

An obstruction causes dilatation of those parts of the urinary tract that are situated more proximally. If it persists, eventually it will lead to total func-tional failure. Obstruction of the renal tubules leads to acute renal failure.

Obstruction to the renal pelvis and calices causes "hydronephrosis," in which there is progressive enlargement of the calices and pelvis, leading to thinning of the renal cortex. If this persists, the glomeruli cease to function. Unless relieved, the damage becomes permanent, with ultimate complete renal failure. If there is obstruction of the bladder or the bladder neck, the bladder will dilate. If of long standing, trabeculation (hypertrophy of the bladder muscle) and diverticula develop; if the vesicoureteric orifices become incompetent there is dilatation of the ureters and bilateral hydronephroses.

The clinical manifestations of an obstruction vary, depending on its cause and how long it has been present. Of great importance is the risk of superimposed infection, as stagnant urine is a fertile breeding ground for bacteria.

Radiography plays a very important role in the diagnosis of both stones and obstruction. Calcified calculi may be seen on plain films, and the IVP gives invaluable information concerning the nature and level of the obstruction and its effect on the renal tract proximally.

Neoplasms of the Kidney

Benign

True benign neoplasms of the kidney are rare and uncommonly seen on radiography; they present as space-occupying lesions. A rare lesion is "angiomyolipoma." Radiography is important in the diagnosis of this tumor, as it contains much fat, which appears as radiotranslucencies; it also is highly vascular, which can be demonstrated by angiography.

"Solitary cysts" are common in adults and probably occur in more than half of the population over the age of 50 years. It is thought that they are acquired lesions and not true neoplasms. They usually are single and commonly are found in a lower pole of a kidney, although multiple ones are not unknown. Their fluid content is very similar to urine. On IVP, they are seen as masses displacing the calices and distorting the renal outline. Their cystic nature can be shown by both CT scanning and ultrasound. They may be demonstrated by contrast material injected at percutaneous cyst puncture. Angiography shows them to be avascular. There are diagnostic problems in differentiating these cysts from the more sinister malignant tumors.

Malignant

ADENOCARCINOMA OF THE KIDNEY (ALSO KNOWN AS HYPERNEPHROMA, CLEAR CELL CARCINOMA, OR GRAWITZ TUMOR). Most of the malignant tumors seen radiographically are of this type. Their incidence increases in people past the age of 40 years, being twice as frequent in men as in women. Adenocarcinomas often present as hematuria; hence, the patients are referred for an IVP. A space-occupying mass is shown on the IVP and this reflects the nature of these tumors. They usually are large, roundish, tend to break through the renal capsule, and, because of their unusually rapid growth, often have necrotic centers. Further investigation includes ultrasound or CT scans followed by angiography. Since they usually are highly vascular, the angiogram will show a tumor circulation, sometimes with an avascular center due to the necrosis.

These tumors metastasize readily. They are unusual in that there often is metastatic growth into the renal veins and the inferior vena cava, which may be shown on venography. Blood-borne metastases reach the lungs, giving rise to multiple rounded shadows. Metastases may also occur to other organs; e.g., liver, bone.

NEPHROBLASTOMA (WILMS' TUMOR). This is a malignant tumor of childhood, almost invariably developing before the age of five years. Unlike the adenocarcinoma, it has an equal sex incidence. Often these children present with evidence of a mass only, felt by the mother when bathing the child. IVP shows a huge abdominal mass, with the kidney grossly displaced. If not treated, these tumors show evidence of widespread metastases to areas such as lung, liver, and lymph nodes. The original poor prognosis has been much improved by modern treatment with radiotherapy and cytotoxic drugs.

CARCINOMA OF THE RENAL PELVIS. This is a tumor of the transitional epithelium and is much less common than the adenocarcinoma. It grows as a mass into the renal pelvis or sometimes in a major calix. It may block the calices or the pelviureteric junction. Radiography will show these features of the lesion. Metastases usually are local, distant ones being uncommon and appearing late in the course of the disease.

Tumors of the ureter are rare but have the same features as those of the renal pelvis.

Neoplasms of the Bladder

Benign

These are uncommon. Papillomatous growths are the most frequent, but all are potentially malignant if not treated.

Malignant

CARCINOMA OF THE BLADDER.   This usually is seen after the age of 50 years and its incidence is three times higher in men than in women. Its etiology has been related to such factors as smoking, excessive coffee drinking, and the industrial use of certain aniline dyes.

Cystoscopy is the method of choice for the diagnosis of these tumors. However, as these patients frequently present with hematuria, an IVP often is the first method of investigation and it may show the tumor. Occasionally the radiographer is asked to perform a cystogram to define the extent of the tumor, which may be difficult for the cystoscopist to assess if it is enormous. Distant metastases of bladder carcinoma develop late, but local invasion is more common and occurs earlier. If the tumor is situated close to a vesicoureteric orifice, the orifice is invaded by the neoplasm, leading to obstruction of the ureter and eventually failure of that kidney. The tumor may also spread directly through the bladder wall, involving pelvic structures.

Tumors of the urethra are rare, but carcinomas do occur occasionally.

6 / GENITAL SYSTEMS
(Including Pregnancy)

Male Genital Tract

Prostate

BENIGN HYPERPLASIA, a common lesion in men over the age of 50 years, is due to hormonal changes associated with aging. As the prostate completely surrounds the proximal urethra, this hyperplasia often interferes with bladder emptying. Micturition difficulties result, including chronic obstruction. The condition can be relieved either by surgical removal of the whole gland or by a TUR (transurethral resection by passage of an endoscope through the urethra to core out the enlarged gland). Radiography does not play a significant role in the diagnosis of the actual hyperplasia but is very important in demonstrating the obstructive changes; e.g., enlarged bladder, hydronephrosis. The often-obtained postmicturition bladder film is used to demonstrate the presence of any retained urine.

Prostatic calculi are easily recognized on plain films. They are seen as small, multiple calcified shadows in the prostate of many males over the age of 50. They are of no clinical significance.

Adenocarcinoma occurs in males over the age of 50, being the third most common carcinoma of males. It does not appear to be related to benign hyperplasia. Radiography plays little or no role in the diagnosis of the primary tumor but is important in demonstrating many of the features of the spread of the disease. The carcinoma may invade the adjacent pelvic tissues, and an IVP may show obstruction of the ureters by the neoplasm. Skeletal metastases are common, eventually developing in at least 75% of all patients. The metastases are unusual because most of them are osteoblastic, i.e., they produce dense sclerotic shadows in the bone x-rays, unlike most other metastases, which are osteolytic, destroying bone. The disease is controlled by hormonal therapy; e.g., oral estrogens, orchidectomy (castration); if successful, this produces increased sclerosis of the bony metastases.

Testes

Diseases of the testes are of little importance to radiographers, with the exception of malignant tumors, which are rare. The *seminoma* usually occurs between ages 30 and 40 years. It has an excellent prognosis because it is very sensitive to radiation therapy. The *teratoma* occurs at about the same age but has a much worse prognosis. Radiography plays little part in the initial diagnosis of these primary tumors but is important in demonstrating their metastases. Lymphangiography and CT scanning may be used to show enlarged nodes, but remember that the lymph drainage of the testes is to the upper para-aortic nodes. Metastases also occur to the lung and liver.

Female Genital Tract

Congenital Anomalies

The uterine cavity may be divided partially (bicornuate) or completely into two chambers. This abnormality may affect the course of pregnancy, leading to abortion. Hysterosalpingography may be performed in patients with recurrent abortions to exclude the possibility of such a congenital anomaly.

Cervix

CARCINOMA. The incidence of this carcinoma is very high, second only in frequency to breast. It nearly always develops in parous women (those who have borne children). Radiography usually plays no role in the diagnosis of the primary tumor but is important in demonstrating some of the metastatic spread. This may be local and affect the urinary tract, causing obstruction at various levels. Spread may be into the iliac and aortic lymph nodes, and lymphangiography can demonstrate this. Later in the course of the disease, distant metastases develop and can be demonstrated by examinations such as chest x-rays and CT scanning of the liver.

Other diseases of the cervix such as cervicitis are of no importance to radiographers.

Uterine Body

The conditions of radiographic importance are neoplasms.

FIBROID. This is a benign tumor of the smooth muscle (leiomyoma). It develops as a solid round mass in the wall of the uterus and may protrude from its external surface or into its lumen. Fibroids often are multiple, and hysterosalpingography can aid in their detection. Small ones may interfere with pregnancy either by causing miscarriages or obstructing labor. They regress after the menopause, some undergoing calcification; thus, they may be detected by chance in elderly women by a plain pelvic x-ray showing a roundish, densely calcified mass.

CARCINOMA. Its incidence is much lower than carcinoma of the cervix and usually occurs in nulliparous women (those who have not borne children). The main role of radiography is to demonstrate metastases, and this tumor behaves in the same way as carcinoma of the cervix.

(Endometrial tissue [uterine glands] occasionally is found in an abnormal site outside the uterus. This is called "endometriosis" and is of little significance to the radiographer. Rarely, this aberrant endometrial tissue invades the wall of the adjacent gut, either large or small, and may simulate carcinoma.)

Ovaries

Benign cysts of different types are quite common and, if of sufficient size, present on a plain x-ray film as a pelvic soft tissue mass. Of particular interest to the radiographer is the teratoma, sometimes called the *dermoid cyst*. This cyst, derived from the ectodermal tissues, often contains teeth visible on plain films. It also frequently contains fatty material and, therefore, may appear radiolucent.

Malignant neoplasms of the ovary are of little importance to radiographers. An unusual secondary neoplasm is the "Krukenberg tumor," which is a metastasis from a carcinoma of the stomach implanted into the ovaries.

Fallopian Tubes

One of the causes of female infertility is blockage of the tubes due to adhesions from previous infection (salpingitis). Hysterosalpingography may be used to demonstrate this by failure of the contrast material to spill into the peritoneal cavity. Sometimes, after acute salpingitis has subsided, a fluid collection is left in the distended tube (hydrosalpinx) and this can be demonstrated by hysterosalpingography. One of the complications of chronic infection of the tubes is the liability of the fertilized ovum to become implanted in an extrauterine situation, giving rise to an *ectopic pregnancy*.

Pregnancy

Pregnancy is associated with many important changes in the body of the mother, and modifies many maternal diseases. Most of these are of little importance to the radiographer, but the effects on the renal tract are of interest. In the rare cases where an IVP is performed during pregnancy, varying degrees of dilatation of the renal tract may be seen. There are three causes for this. First, pregnancy is associated with considerable changes in the hormonal state of the mother. These cause some relaxation of smooth muscle, including that in the ureteric wall. Second, as the fetus grows, the uterus presses on the pelvic brim, causing partial mechanical obstruction of the ureters at this level. Finally, dilatation may be due to infection in the upper renal tract.

Toxemia of Pregnancy

This can develop in the late stages of pregnancy, causing proteinuria and hypertension. Its causes are obscure but probably are related to changes in the kidneys. Seriously affected patients may go on to have convulsions (eclampsia), and premature labor may be precipitated. There are no radiographic changes associated with this condition, but if the patient is being x-rayed, the radiographer should understand the serious nature of the mother's illness.

Tubal Pregnancy

Instead of the fertilized ovum implanting in the body of the uterus, it may implant in an abnormal or ectopic site, usually the fallopian tube. As the pregnancy develops, the placental tissues erode through the tubal wall and then rupture, usually with acute bleeding, into the peritoneal cavity. These patients, therefore, often present as an "acute abdomen." Plain radiography has little to offer in the diagnosis, but ultrasound can be a useful diagnostic tool.

Rarely, the pregnancy terminates without rupture. If it is not removed, it may go on to calcify and be visible on an x-ray film as a "lithopedion."

Placenta Previa

Instead of the placenta being implanted in its normal position in the upper half of the uterus, usually on the posterior wall, it develops in the lower half of the uterus. The closer the placenta is to the internal os the more likelihood there is of complications, such as bleeding, during pregnancy. If the placenta actually covers the os there will be obstruction of labor. If this lesion is suspected clinically, various imaging techniques may be used to display it. Angiography and isotope scans have been used in the past, but the method of choice today is ultrasound scanning.

Multiple Pregnancies

Twins occur in approximately one in 88 pregnancies. Of these, about one-third are "monovular" (from the same fertilized ovum, giving rise to identical twins) and the other two-thirds are "biovular." Triplets and quadruplets are much rarer. Multiple pregnancies have an increased incidence of complications for both the mother and the fetuses because of the liabilities of premature birth and of a lower birth weight. Diagnosis of this condition, therefore, is important, and either plain film radiography or ultrasound scanning can be used to confirm or exclude the diagnosis if suspected clinically.

Abnormalities of the Amniotic Fluid

The amniotic fluid is formed partly by excretion from the amnion and partly in the latter stages of pregnancy by the fetal urine. Reabsorption takes place by the fetal swallowing of the fluid and subsequent excretion back across the placenta into the maternal circulation. There is, therefore, a continuous circulation of fluid.

Rarely there may be a decrease in the amount of amniotic fluid (oligohydramnios). This usually is due to a failure of fetal urine formation such as occurs if the fetal kidneys have failed to develop or if there is total obstruction of the fetal urinary tract. More commonly there is an excess of amniotic fluid (polyhydramnios). This may be due to interference with the swallowing and absorption mechanisms of the fetus; e.g., tracheoesophageal fistula, duodenal atresia. The occurrence of polyhydramnios will alert the clinician to the possible need for radiographic investigation of the neonate to exclude abnormalities such as these.

Obstructed Labor

Delivery of the fetus may be hindered by many different causes, including failure of the uterine muscle. There are a number of *mechanical* causes; e.g., abnormalities of fetal presentation, narrowing of pelvic diameters (contracted pelvis), uterine fibroids. Radiography, e.g., pelvimetry can be of great value in assessing or excluding these mechanical factors.

Fetal Abnormalities

Commonly, the fetus presents by the vertex (head), but this is not always so. The most common abnormal presentation is by the breech (buttocks). Sometimes the fetus may lie transversely or present by the face or brow. These abnormalities in position are associated with increased fetal mortality, and their assessment by plain film radiography and ultrasound therefore is important.

A number of abnormalities of the fetus can also be detected by both plain film radiography and ultrasound. The most common of these probably would be "anencephaly," where the brain and vault of the skull fail to develop. Sometimes there is gross enlargement of the ventricles of the brain and therefore of the skull, giving rise to "hydro-cephalus."

"Erythroblastosis fetalis" is an uncommon disease in which there is destruction of the fetal red blood cells. It is due to incompatibility of the fetal red blood cells containing an antigen, the Rh factor, with antibodies in the maternal circulation. In severe cases, the fetus becomes edematous and adopts a rather strange posture. These findings sometimes can be seen on plain film radiography or by ultrasound.

Fetal Death

A fetus may die late in pregnancy. This death may be related to diseases of the mother, e.g., hypertension; of the placenta, e.g., infarction; or of the fetus itself, e.g., erythroblastosis. Absent fetal movements indicate to the mother and her obstetrician that death has occurred, but radiography may be used to confirm this. The earliest radiographic change is the detection of free gas in the fetal vessels, usually in the first 48 hours after death. Subsequently, the fetus collapses and this is best seen with overlapping skull bones due to reduction in the volume of the brain (Spalding's sign).

Hydatidiform Mole

This placental lesion is seen in about one in 2,500 pregnancies. Early in pregnancy, the placental tissue fails to develop normally; it becomes cystic and the fetus consequently dies. However, the "pregnancy" continues, with very rapid enlargement of the uterus. If a mole is suspected clinically, plain film radiography or ultrasound scanning will confirm the large soft tissue mass due to the enlarged uterus with no evidence of fetal parts.

Breast

The frequent occurrence of carcinoma of the breast has led to great interest in methods of detecting it in its early stages so that cure may be achieved. Radiographically, this has led to the refinement of soft tissue examinations of the breast by such techniques as plain film mammography, xerography, and ultrasound. The radiographer, therefore, should have some idea of the various tumors that may be found in the breast.

Dysplasias

This group of conditions is due to hormonal imbalance and therefore is bilateral. There are areas of disordered epithelium leading to cyst formation with surrounding reactive fibrosis, so that affected breasts contain palpable lumps. There always is the problem that there may be an associated occult carcinoma. Mammography will demonstrate the diffuse involvement of both breasts by the cysts and fibrosis whereas ultrasound is valuable in confirmation of the cysts.

Benign Neoplasms

By far the most common is "fibroadenoma." It is a well-defined rounded mass, usually small and solitary, without any infiltration of the surrounding breast tissue. These features can be shown by mammography.

Carcinoma

It is estimated that one in 16 of all women develops this neoplasm, and it is responsible for about one-fifth of all female deaths from carcinoma. Although it also occurs in the male, it is much rarer. It is known that at least 5% of all women with carcinoma in one breast subsequently will develop it in the other. The neoplasm often is seen on mammography as a dense mass infiltrating the surrounding breast tissue. It is irregular in outline due to fibrotic reaction. In advanced cases, this fibrosis leads to pulling in of the nipple (retraction). In nearly half of the cases, numerous areas of microcalcification can be detected, and these are very typical of breast carcinoma.

Carcinoma of the breast metastasizes initially via the lymphatic system, with involvement of the axillary nodes. Blood-borne metastases also occur and may develop in many organs; e.g., lungs, liver, bone. Treatment of the metastases is by either deep x-ray therapy, cytotoxic drugs, or hormones. If these therapies are successful, metastases in the lung may cease to grow or will regress whereas lytic metastases in bone may undergo sclerosis.

(Paget's disease of the nipple is a premalignant condition. It should not be confused with Paget's disease of bone.)

7 / SKELETAL SYSTEM

ORGAN IMAGING plays a vital role in the diagnosis of diseases of bones and joints. Because bones contain calcium, they are visualized on plain films. More recently, CT scanning has provided extra information in selected cases. Isotope scanning also has proved to be of considerable value, as areas of increased bone activity are readily detected. Often, isotope examinations show evidence of disease before there are changes on plain films.

Trauma

Fractures

A "fracture" is defined as a discontinuity of a bone due to mechanical forces. It may be caused in two ways. There may be application of force *directly* to the bone or, alternatively, the force may be transmitted *indirectly* along the line of the bone (e.g., Colles' fracture of the radius due to a fall on an outstretched hand).

There are many different types of fractures, and the following terms are used to describe them.

Simple fracture—the bone is divided into two parts only.

Comminuted fracture—the bone is divided into three or more parts.

Impacted fracture—the cortical bone is jammed or telescoped into the cancellous bone. A "compression fracture" of a vertebral body is an impaction injury, usually due to excessive flexion.

Fissure fracture—there is an incomplete crack through the bone.

Greenstick fracture—there is a fissure fracture, with bending of the bone on its convex side only. This type is seen only in children's bones, which are elastic.

Stress fracture—there is excessive overuse of a bone. The classic example is the "march fracture" seen in the metatarsals of army recruits who do unaccustomed marching. Often a fracture line is not visible on early x-ray of a stress fracture, although increased isotope uptake will indicate a lesion. Later, its presence can be deduced by the appearance of a small amount of new bone formation (periostitis) at the site.

Pathologic fracture—a fracture occurs through an area of already-diseased bone.

Compound fracture—the skin or a mucosal surface is pierced by the ends of a fractured bone.

Fracture Union

Breaking of a bone causes local tissue damage and considerable hemorrhage. This leads to inflammation and the formation of fibrous tissue. Osteoblastic cells, mainly from the periosteum, convert this tissue into bone. This is called "callus" and can be seen on plain films. As the repair process continues, the callus becomes incorporated into the ends of the fractured bone, restoring the strength of the bone (consolidation). Subsequent activity by osteoblasts and osteoclasts restores the shape of the bone to normal (remodeling). This may be incomplete if the fracture unites with marked deformity.

Movement between ends of a fractured bone interferes with these processes. Hence, immobilization (e.g., by external plaster casts or internal nails) is essential for union. Other factors such as increasing age, poor diet, and the presence of disease will retard union.

A fracture that has failed to unite with bony callus is said to show "nonunion." The fractured ends are held together by fibrous tissue. Movement may lead to sclerosis of the bone ends, with the development of a false joint (pseudarthrosis).

Complications of Fractures

Infection. This is particularly likely to occur with a compound fracture and will delay union.

Injuries to other structures. The ends of the fractured bones may damage adjacent structures; e.g., a fractured rib penetrating the lung, causing a pneumothorax; damage to the brachial artery and the median nerve in front of the elbow, complicating a supracondylar fracture of the humerus.

Calcification and ossification. If there is extensive soft tissue damage around a fracture, with much bleeding from the fracture, as the fracture unites there may be excessive calcification, leading to ossification in the surrounding muscles (myositis ossificans). Fractures around the elbow joint are prone to this complication.

Fat embolism. Occasionally, when there is severe fracturing of a major bone such as the femur, fat from the bone marrow enters the circulation and causes embolization of various organs. This condition may be detected on chest x-ray when a blotchy appearance is seen in the lungs. Fat embolism of the brain may result in the death of the patient. Patients with extensive fat embolism are seriously ill.

Sudeck's atrophy. There is gross exaggeration of the osteoporosis that normally occurs with the immobilization of a fracture, but the cause is obscure. Because of the much greater loss of calcium than usual, it may be difficult to obtain satisfactory films of the area, especially if it still is immobilized in plaster.

Battered Babies

This unfortunate condition is seen in children under the age of three years who have been subjected to severe and repeated physical abuse, usually by one parent only. The amount of physical abuse may be sufficient to cause permanent damage to the child, and it is thought that up to 10% of these children die as a direct result of the trauma. Radiography plays an important role in the detection of this condition. Multiple fractures, often in the metaphyseal areas, will be demonstrated in various stages of healing. Subdural hemorrhage also is a common finding and should be suspected if skull fractures are demonstrated. It is thought that up to a quarter of these children suffer permanent brain damage due to the subdural hematomas.

Spondylolisthesis

There is anterior subluxation of the body of L-5 on the sacrum. This is due to defects in the neural arch of L-5 between the articular facets (pars interarticularis). Special oblique views or tomography may be needed to demonstrate the defects. There is dispute as to the cause of this condition. Some authorities maintain that it is a congenital anomaly, but much evidence points to it being a stress fracture. Occasionally it is seen at higher levels of the lumbar spine.

It is a cause of low back pain. It does not produce neurologic signs unless the degree of slipping is so marked that there is traction on the cauda equina.

Congenital Defects

There are innumerable developmental anomalies of the skeleton that are readily shown by plain film radiography. Some of the defects cause widespread disturbances throughout the skeleton, but many are localized to one or a few areas.

Many of the localized anomalies are of little significance, being hardly more than "normal variants." Examples of this type include the accessory epiphysis at the base of the fifth metatarsal, the division of the sesamoid bone beneath the head of the first metatarsal into two or four parts, and the occurrence of a small bone at the posterior tubercle of the talus—"os trigonum." Of more clinical significance are developmental anomalies such as "cervical ribs"; these are a pair of ribs arising from the seventh cervical vertebra, which may interfere with the nerves and vessels to the upper limbs. Another common site for anomalies is the lumbosacral junction, where L-5 may show partial or total fusion with the sacrum (sacralization). This condition usually is referred to as "transitional lumbosacral vertebra" and may cause backache and sciatica. More severe local deformities exist, even to a partial or complete failure of development of various parts of the limb bones. A well-known example of this is the interference with limb development that occurred in fetuses born to mothers who had taken thalidomide during pregnancy.

The two most common generalized defects will be described, both of them being inherited.

Osteogenesis Imperfecta

There is failure of the skeleton to ossify properly. The bones are slender, with thin cortices, and very prone to fracture. In severe cases, multiple fractures occur in utero. During childhood, these patients run the risk of fracturing bones on trivial trauma. From the radiographer's point of view, it often is difficult to obtain satisfactory films of these fractured limbs through plaster because of the underdevelopment (poor calcification) of the bones. These children often are deaf.

Achondroplasia

The preosseous cartilage fails to develop properly, interfering with ossification. This leads to considerable reduction in the length of the limbs, so that these patients become dwarfs. The base of the skull also is affected but the vault is not because it develops from membrane, not cartilage. There is involvement of the vertebral column, including narrowing of the vertebral canal, which can lead to neurologic complications in adult life. Despite their short limbs, achondroplastic dwarfs have normal-sized bodies. They are of normal intelligence and often find employment in circuses.

Infective Lesions

Infection of bone is known as "osteomyelitis." This usually is caused by organisms arriving via the bloodstream, but uncommonly it is due to direct infection; e.g., compound fracture. Although the disease may occur at any age, its greatest incidence is in children.

Patients with *acute* osteomyelitis are extremely ill. The common site for the disease is in the limbs, especially in the metaphyses around the knee joint. The inflammatory reaction rapidly causes a rise in pressure within the bone, which is constricted by its periosteum so that there is compression and thrombosis of its vessels. This leads to death of the bone, usually within 24–48 hours. Unfortunately, these changes cannot be appreciated on plain x-ray films. After the bone has died there will be attempts at repair, and it is not until about 14 days that sufficient calcium has been removed and new periosteal bone laid down for radiographic evidence of this condition to be evident. Therefore, the condition must be diagnosed on clinical grounds and treated early with antibiotics and local drainage.

If the treatment is delayed or inadequate, the bone dies; this piece of dead bone is known as a "sequestrum." The term "involucrum" refers to the new bone that is laid down around the sequestrated bone. If treatment is inadequate, the condition becomes *chronic* and other complications such as abscess formation and a skin sinus will follow. The reaction of the bone to this persisting infection causes marked sclerosis; therefore, the radiographer may need to overexpose the films or use tomography to demonstrate sequestra hidden within the area. If the infection occurs insidiously, a chronic osteomyelitis develops, localized in the bone in a circumscribed fashion (Brodie's abscess).

Tuberculous infection of bone now is a rare condition in Western communities. It is a chronic process, usually associated with considerable osteoporosis and bone destruction. Infection of the vertebral column involves the *disks* rather than the vertebral bodies. Tuberculosis of the lower thoracic and lumbar vertebral disks, if not treated, gives rise to abscesses tracking along the psoas muscle;

these may be seen as ill-defined masses of calcification. When the infection is treated successfully, healing occurs by bony fusion (ankylosis).

Metabolic Bone Disease

In this group of generalized diseases there is disturbance of the physiologic processes responsible for the maintenance of normal bone, so that the bone becomes weakened and prone to fracture. By definition, lesions such as infections and neoplasms are excluded.

Osteoporosis

In this condition there is a lack of osteoid, so that insufficient bone is formed, although what is formed is properly ossified. There are many causes for this, but radiographically they usually cannot be differentiated.

SENILE OSTEOPOROSIS. This is the most common form. It is seen in people over the age of 45 years and in women more than in men. It sometimes is referred to as "postmenopausal osteoporosis." Its etiology is obscure, but causes postulated include hormonal imbalance, defective nutrition, and lessening physical activity. The radiographic changes mirror the pathologic ones, so that x-ray films show loss of calcium from the skeleton, with thinning of the cortices and lessening of the number of trabeculae. As the bone becomes progressively weakened there is evidence of fracturing, often in the vertebral bodies, and eventually the patient may develop marked kyphosis, with diminished height. Patients with advanced disease suffer considerable pain, and the condition is difficult to treat.

ENDOCRINE DISEASES. In some of these there is disturbance of calcium metabolism so that this is lost from the body and, therefore, the skeleton in excessive amounts. The best known are "hyperparathyroidism" and "Cushing's disease." The administration of cortisone and other steroid drugs can mimic these conditions and, therefore, are examples of iatrogenic disease.

PROLONGED IMMOBILIZATION. If the patient or any part of the patient (limb in plaster following fracture) is immobilized for any length of time, the part or parts lose calcium because of the lack of the stimulus of normal activity. This osteoporosis in an immobilized limb can cause radiographic problems because the lessened calcium content makes it more difficult to obtain an adequate radiographic shadow.

Osteomalacia

In this condition there is a normal amount of osteoid but, due to lack of calcium, it is defectively ossified. Osteomalacia is rare in Western communities and usually is secondary to some other disease; e.g., malabsorption from the small bowel. However, on a world-wide basis, defective nutrition, especially inadequate intakes of vitamin D and calcium, would be the main cause. As the bones are deficient in calcium, they are soft, leading to bowing, with incomplete fractures (Looser's zones) appearing later.

Rickets

Classic rickets is a disease of infants and early childhood in which the cartilage fails to ossify properly due to lack of vitamin D. Therefore, it is a variety of osteomalacia. The softness of the bones leads to deformities such as bowlegs. If severe and not treated, it will cause deformities of the pelvis, which may be of considerable importance in females when they reach the age of childbearing. It now is extremely rare in Australia because even if vitamin D is lacking in the diet, the skin, on exposure to sunlight, is able to make sufficient vitamin D to compensate for this.

A similar condition may be seen in children affected by chronic renal disease sufficient to cause lowering of the serum calcium. This is referred to as "renal rickets," and in Australia and other Western communities is more common than the dietary form, although it still is rare.

Paget's Disease

Paget's disease (osteitis deformans) occurs in people over the age of 40 years and is more common in men than in women. Its cause is not known and it may affect one or several bones. The bones involved most frequently are pelvis, lumbar spine, femora, skull, and tibias. Initially, the bone is softened by excessive activity of osteoclasts removing calcium. This progresses at varying speeds until most or the whole of a bone is affected. Due to the softening there often is bowing of the bone, especially if it is in the lower limb, and there also may be fractures. There is some displacement of the periosteum so that the bone eventually becomes slightly enlarged. Later, repair occurs, with sclerotic new bone laid down in the areas of absorption. Usually these processes are simultaneous so that an x-ray shows mixed areas of osteolysis and osteosclerosis in an enlarged bone. This enlargement may lead to narrowing of various areas, e.g., the dorsal vertebral canal, with consequent pressure effects on the spinal cord leading to paraplegia. A rare complication of Paget's disease is malignant degeneration, with the development of a sarcoma.

Bone Infarction

A sudden interruption of the blood supply to a bone will result in bone death by infarction (aseptic necrosis). Of particular interest to radiographers is the occurrence of this condition in growing epiphyses of children. The reasons for this are not entirely clear, but it appears to be due to repeated trauma of a relatively mild degree. The condition is seen in many epiphyses; the time of involvement of each epiphysis varies, apparently being related to the most rapid growth phase of that particular epiphysis, when it is more vulnerable to injury. These conditions usually are referred to as "osteochondritis," but there often is a specific name for each individual epiphysis; e.g., Perthe's disease of the hip, Osgood-Schlatter's disease of the tibial tubercle. X-rays of the affected area initially show density due to the death of the bone. The epiphysis then undergoes fragmentation. Next, there is invasion by granulation tissue, causing lytic areas. Ultimately, this is followed by repair when normal bone is again laid down. The exact effect on any particular epiphysis depends on a number of factors, especially the normal stresses to which that particular one is subjected. Some repair without residual deformity whereas others, especially the hip, may end up with deformed joint surfaces, leading to early osteoarthritis.

Bone infarction is much rarer in adults. It follows certain fractures, such as subcapital fractures of the femoral neck and fractures through the waist of the scaphoid when there is interference with the blood supply to the minor fragments. It may complicate some types of hemolytic anemia, e.g., sickle cell disease, where the arteries are blocked by clumping of the abnormal red cells. Aseptic necrosis of bone may also follow embolization of the bone marrow by gas bubbles ("the bends"), and this occurs in people who have been subjected to greatly increased atmospheric pressures; e.g., divers. If decompression is too rapid, gas bubbles form in the blood and block the vessels in the bone marrow. There are no radiographic changes for the acute stage, but if the embolization is widespread there is necrosis of the weight-bearing ends of the bones, with eventual crumbling of the articular surfaces leading to severe osteoarthritis.

Neoplasms

Neoplasms may arise in bone or cartilage. (Neoplasms of the bone marrow are described in the section on the Reticuloendothelial System.)

Benign Neoplasms

OSTEOMA. This is a true but rare neoplasm of osteoid tissue. Most lesions are in the bones of the skull and nasal sinuses. X-rays will show a lesion with a well-organized bony structure, often protruding into a sinus. Osteomas are of little clinical significance.

OSTEOCHONDROMA (EXOSTOSIS). This common neoplasm is due to a localized overgrowth of bone. This gives a bony projection of varying size, on the distal part of which is a small cap of cartilage. While the skeleton is growing, the osteochondroma will increase in size, but this usually stops about the age of puberty. Radiography will show the bony projection often near a major joint, especially the knee. In themselves, these tumors are of little significance, although they may interfere with joint movement or press on adjacent structures such as skin or nerves.

OSTEOID OSTEOMA. This rare tumor of bone produces excessively dense sclerotic bone around a small area of cartilage. It occurs chiefly in the lower limb bones of young adults. Radiographic demonstration of this may necessitate overexposed films or tomography. The condition may be confused with a Brodie's abscess.

CHONDROMA (ENCHONDROMA). This tumor may develop anywhere in the skeleton where cartilage is present. Most chondromas occur in the small bones of the hands and feet, and patients are x-rayed either because of swelling or of pain due to a pathologic fracture through the lesion. Malignant degeneration is rare but is more likely to occur in chondromas of flat bones; e.g., pelvis.

GIANT CELL TUMOR (OSTEOCLASTOMA). This tumor of young adults is seen in the distal ends of the long bones, especially around the knee and in the distal end of the radius. It extends to the joint surface but does not break through it. There is extensive removal of bone from the area of the tumor, so that superficially it may resemble a malignancy. However, most are benign and can be removed surgically. If the osteoclastoma recurs there is an increasing risk of it becoming malignant.

Malignant Neoplasms

METASTASES. Secondary malignancies of bone are much more common than primary tumors. On x-ray, most metastases show evidence of bone destruction. However, carcinoma of the prostate nearly always has metastases with some or much sclerosis. With the exception of the prostate there is no means of telling the primary from which the metastases came, but the most frequent sites are breast, lung, gastrointestinal tract, and kidney.

OSTEOGENIC SARCOMA. This rare primary bone neoplasm usually occurs in late adolescence. Although it may develop anywhere in the skeleton, the vast majority of cases occur at the ends of long bones, especially around the knee. This lesion is highly malignant. X-rays demonstrate this with evidence of extensive bone destruction, a mass in the adjacent soft tissues, and new bone formation. Metastases occur early, especially to the lungs, as these tumors are highly vascular. Sometimes the condition can be confused clinically with acute osteomyelitis because the tumor is painful and may resemble an inflammatory lesion. The prognosis is not good, and most patients die within five years.

There is another form of primary osteogenic sarcoma occurring much later in life as a complication of Paget's disease. This is rapidly fatal, most patients dying within a few months of diagnosis.

CHONDROSARCOMA. This malignancy of cartilage appears later in life, usually about the age of 45 years. More than half of the cases occur in pelvic bones. Chondrosarcomas give rise to large tumor masses often containing areas of calcification and ossification. The tumor runs a much more benign course than the osteogenic sarcomas, patients often surviving for many years.

Joints

Diseases of synovial joints are of considerable importance, being responsible for much morbidity. There are many different causes for them, some not completely understood. "Arthritis" is any inflammatory lesion of a joint, and may be acute or chronic.

Trauma

There may be *direct* injury to a joint; alternatively, there may be an application of *indirect* force; e.g., tearing of the semilunar cartilage of the knee by twisting. Complete and persistent displacement between the articular surface of one bone and that of its fellow is a "dislocation." A "subluxation" is a partial dislocation. A "sprain" is temporary subluxation, with the bones returning to normal alignment. Plain films will demonstrate the malalignment of the bones and any associated fractures. Fluid in a joint is an "effusion." Blood in a joint is a "hemarthrosis."

Infection

Most infections are acute, being due to bloodborne spread of organisms such as the *Staphylococcus*, more rarely the gonococcus. The joint becomes very painful, with evidence of acute inflammation. If the condition is not treated there is destruction of the cartilage, leading to joint narrowing. Ultimately, repair occurs, with bony ankylosis of the joint leading to a fixed deformity. In the initial stages, x-ray will show little change apart from an effusion, but after ten to 14 days there will be osteoporosis of the surrounding bones. Later films will demonstrate the joint narrowing and ultimately the ankylosis.

Chronic infections of joints, such as tuberculosis, now are rare in Western communities.

Rheumatoid Arthritis

The cause of this is not known, although it is thought to be an autoimmune disease. Classically, it is a chronic condition with recurrent acute phases, although sometimes only one or two attacks occur without long-term sequelae. It usually commences in middle life and is three times more common in women than in men. An inflammatory reaction develops in the joint, with thickening of the synovial tissues (pannus), which then causes destruction of the joint surfaces by pressure. It commonly affects, at least initially, the small joints of the hands and the feet, tending to be bilateral and symmetric. In severe cases, many joints, including those of the vertebral column, may be involved. If not treated, it leads to marked joint destruction with considerable deformity. Radiologically there is initial osteoporosis with soft tissue swelling around the affected joints. As the condition progresses, x-rays show narrowing of the joints, erosions of the ends of the adjacent bones, and the eventual development of joint narrowing with gross deformities.

Infrequently, the upper cervical vertebrae may be involved, with destruction of the atlantoaxial joint. This leads to instability, which may be demonstrated radiologically by flexion and extension laterals.

Ankylosing Spondylitis

This nearly always starts in the sacroiliac joints, but may spread later to involve the vertebral column and, rarely, adjacent major joints. Initially there is an inflammatory reaction in the sacroiliac joints, which proceeds to complete bony fusion of these joints, a radiographic hallmark of the condition. If the spine is involved, ossification develops in the longitudinal ligaments, giving rise to the radiographic appearance of "bamboo spine." The vertebral bodies thus are fused to each other and many of the advanced cases have a fixed gross kyphosis. There may be involvement of the costovertebral joints, leading to respiratory embarrassment and, as a result, in severe cases many patients die of pulmonary disease. Occasionally, patients with ankylosing spondylitis show evidence of other autoimmune diseases; e.g., iritis, ulcerative colitis, pulmonary fibrosis.

Osteoarthritis

This is a very common degenerative disease of the synovial joints. Any joint may be involved, but those subjected to much use are more likely to be affected; e.g., distal interphalangeal of fingers. This is "fair wear and tear," but sometimes there has been overstressing; e.g., knees in obese people, previous severe joint disease.

X-ray initially shows narrowing of the joint due to the loss of articular cartilage, the basic lesion of osteoarthritis. This loss results in the underlying bone becoming sclerotic as a reaction to the unusual stress. There is formation of extra buttresses of bone around the joint margins (lipping). Other changes that may develop are the formation of "loose bodies" within the joint and of "subarticular cysts" due to the pumping of synovial fluid through the fragmented cartilage into the underlying bone. Eventually there is considerable loss of function, with associated pain. It is this pain and loss of function that cause patients to seek medical advice. In recent years, the development of artificial hips (and other joints) has enabled many of these people to achieve mobility again, with relief from their pain.

Neuropathic Arthritis (Charcot's Joint)

This is a degenerative arthritis in which the changes are grossly exaggerated because the joint has lost sensation, leading to excessive use. The patient is unable to appreciate the damage being done to the joint, so there is severe destruction. The classic cause of the condition was advanced syphilis, but today diabetes is the usual etiology, although it may be seen in some rare diseases of the central nervous system; e.g., syringomyelia.

Plain films will show the gross destructive changes, often with considerable subluxation. The radiographer may be surprised at the patient's lack of symptoms.

Disk Herniation

There is degeneration of the anulus fibrosus around the intervertebral disk so that it undergoes "fracturing." As a result, pressure forces out the nucleus pulposus so that it may press on nerve roots, causing pain, sometimes interfering with function in part of a limb. Long-standing disk herniation is reflected in x-rays as a narrowing of the intervertebral disk; if this is severe there may be sclerosis and lipping of the adjacent vertebral bodies. The herniated nucleus pulposus may be demonstrated by myelography. Diskography is performed occasionally to demonstrate the degenerative changes in the disk.

Gout

This is an inherited metabolic disease, more common in males. Due to defects in the metabolism of nitrogen, excessive uric acid is formed and may be deposited in the soft tissues, such a deposit being a "tophus." Sometimes the uric acid crystals may be laid down in a joint, often the first metatarsophalangeal joint. The condition is extremely painful and the initial attack may be precipitated by some unusual stress; e.g., unrelated surgery. The condition tends to be recurrent, with involvement of other joints. Eventually there is destruction of the articular cartilage so that, on x-ray, appearances resemble that of simple osteoarthritis. However, if calcified tophi can be seen in the soft tissues, the diagnosis can be made radiologically.

Long-term complications may occur in gout. The production of excessive uric acid leads to its increased excretion by the kidneys; hence, the formation of radiolucent stones. Other complications are the development of vascular disease and renal failure due to nephritis.

Hypertrophic Pulmonary Osteoarthropathy

This is a rare condition in which there is painful swelling of the fingers and toes, often involving the wrists and ankles. Radiographically, new bone formation is seen around many of the small and long bones of the limbs. This odd condition is a reaction to a chronic chest condition, nearly always bronchogenic carcinoma. The mechanism of the new bone formation remains a mystery.

8 / CENTRAL NERVOUS SYSTEM

Congenital Lesions

THERE ARE MANY OF THESE, but only those of relevance will be described.

ANENCEPHALY. This is failure of development of the brain and overlying skull vault. Babies born with this defect do not live.

MICROCEPHALY. There is failure of the cerebrum to develop properly, causing a small head.

ARNOLD-CHIARI SYNDROME. This is a rare lesion, with bony fusion of the occiput and the upper cervical vertebrae leading to a small posterior cranial fossa. The medulla, therefore, is forced through the foramen magnum into the upper cervical canal, leading to obstruction of the flow of cerebrospinal fluid. Plain films, CT scanning, and sometimes air studies are used to demonstrate the anatomy of the malformation.

DIASTEMATOMYELIA. There is splitting of the spinal cord into two parts in the sagittal plane so that there is an anterior and posterior horn on each side. Often this is associated with an abnormal midline bony spur, which may be seen on plain films. CT scanning and myelography are used to demonstrate the extent of the lesion.

SPINA BIFIDA. This is a common anomaly due basically to a failure of closure of the developing neural canal, usually caudally. In most instances, this is an isolated abnormality limited to a defect in the neural arch of a vertebra; this is referred to as "spina bifida occulta" and is of no clinical significance. With more extensive defects involving the skin there is protrusion of the coverings of the central nervous system through the defect (meningocele). In a "meningomyelocele" there is protrusion of nerve tissue in addition to the meninges. Depending on the severity of the defect, there will be neurologic deficiencies in the control of the lower limbs, bladder, and rectum. As the central nervous system communicates freely with the exterior, there is risk of infection of the meninges. These unfortunate children are seen frequently in x-ray departments for assessment of their initial defects, for evaluation of their urinary tracts, which often become infected, and for radiographs of their lower limbs, which may be abnormal due to disturbances of innervation.

Hydrocephalus

This is excess cerebrospinal fluid in the cranial cavity. It is accompanied by various degrees of cerebral atrophy, as usually the fluid accumulates in the ventricular system, compressing the brain. If it occurs in the fetus there is great enlargement of the head so that normal delivery of the live infant is impossible.

Hydrocephalus is due to the obstruction of the flow of cerebrospinal fluid. In the *internal* type, this is due to lesions in the aqueduct or in the roof of the fourth ventricle. In the *communicating* type there is external obstruction at the level of the mid-brain where it passes through the opening in the tentorium, so that the ventricular system still is able to communicate with the posterior fossa and spinal canal.

The causes may be either congenital or acquired. The Arnold-Chiari syndrome is an example of *congenital* hydrocephalus. Many infants born with serious degrees of spina bifida also have hydrocephalus. The most common cause of *acquired* hydrocephalus is intracerebral neoplasm. As these tumors grow, they may press on the aqueduct, force the brain stem against the openings of the tentorium, or interfere with the reabsorption of cerebrospinal fluid by the arachnoid granulations. Usually more than one of these mechanisms is at work.

Plain films will show any changes in the bones of the skull, especially in infants. To demonstrate the anatomy of the hydrocephalus more precisely, CT scanning is of great value. Occasionally this needs to be supplemented by contrast studies of the ventricular system by either pneumoencephalography or ventriculography.

Cerebrospinal Fluid Abnormalities

The pressure of the CSF may be increased. This may be due either to an inflammatory lesion of the meninges or to a space-occupying lesion; e.g., cerebral tumor.

The pressure of the CSF may be decreased and this may be precipitous enough to produce little or no flow of CSF on lumbar puncture. This low pressure indicates a block somewhere between the puncture site and the brain, usually caused by a tumor, sometimes by a large prolapsed intervertebral disk.

Fresh blood in the CSF indicates recent bleeding into the subarachnoid space; e.g., from a leaking aneurysm. Sometimes the CSF is yellowish in color (xanthochromia). This indicates old blood in the CSF due to a bleed in the recent past.

Abnormal cells may be found in the CSF, and the nature of these will indicate the underlying lesion; e.g., white blood cells indicate infection. Turbidity of the CSF indicates pus.

Vascular Disorders of the Brain

ANEURYSMS. Small saccular aneurysms may occur on the intracranial vessels. It is not certain if they are congenital. Many of them appear to develop in middle life as a result of atheroma and hypertension, so most probably are acquired. They are symptomless until they rupture (subarachnoid hemorrhage), when the patient experiences a very severe occipital headache and usually becomes comatose, although this may be temporary. Angiography is used to demonstrate the aneurysm. Many of them are on the anterior communicating artery and the major subdivisions of the middle cerebral artery. They are variable in size and shape. Since a significant number of them are multiple, *bilateral* carotid angiography must be done if the patient is being assessed for surgery.

ARTERIOVENOUS MALFORMATIONS. They are congenital lesions with a network of abnormal vessels and may be found anywhere in the brain. They may bleed but are a much less common cause of subarachnoid hemorrhage than are aneurysms. The malformations are supplied by one or more large feeding arteries, with rapid shunting of blood to the venous side, and can be demonstrated by carotid angiography.

CEREBROVASCULAR ACCIDENTS. These commonly are referred to as "strokes." They may be due to *infarction* of the brain or actual *bleeding* into its substance.

Brain infarction is caused by arterial disease, usually thrombosis in an atheromatous vessel. Embolism is rare. Spasm, especially of the small cerebral vessels, also has been suggested as a cause. The atheroma may occur either in vessels within the cranial cavity or at an extracranial site; e.g., origin of the internal carotid artery. As a result of the thrombosis (or embolism), the neurons die, leading to a neurologic deficit (hemiplegia). As the nerve tracts cross over in the brain stem, infarction of the left cerebral hemisphere leads to paralysis of the right side of the body and vice versa. If the degree of neurologic deficit is severe there will be unconsciousness, coma, and ultimately death.

The exact mechanism of bleeding into the brain is not known in most cases, and is presumed to be due to weakness of the vessel wall in the area concerned. The bleeding leads to destruction of neurons and axons, so the clinical picture is very similar to that of infarction.

The advent of CT scanning has made it possible to distinguish between these two conditions in the living patient, and this has greatly influenced the management of these cases. The CT scan in infarction will show a radiolucent area of brain edema, whereas a recent hemorrhage will show as an area of increased density. Should surgery be contemplated to prevent further infarctions, angiography is performed to detect areas of atheroma in the extracranial vessels, including the major vessels of the thorax.

Neoplasms

Most primary neoplasms arise from the supporting neuroglia and not from the neurons. Metastases from neoplasms of the nervous system hardly ever occur outside the central nervous system. There is great variation in the presentation and progress of the various neoplasms, depending on their type and the site at which they occur. In general, the growth of the neoplasm within the rigid bony skull leads to an increase in intracranial pressure. This causes symptoms such as headache, vomiting, and intellectual impairment. Plain skull films may show enlargement of the pituitary fossa, with erosion of the posterior clinoid processes due to the raised pressure. In children, the sutures may be widened (diastasis).

PRIMARY MALIGNANT NEOPLASMS. The "glioma" is the most common, accounting for about half of all brain tumors, and there are several types. The "astrocytoma" is a very slowly growing glioma that usually occurs after the age of 30 years. It is prone to undergo cystic degeneration, and some of these tumors contain calcifications. In contrast, the "glioblastoma" is highly malignant. Similar neoplasms occur in the spinal cord. The "medulloblastoma" is another highly malignant tumor with a very poor prognosis, occurring in the cerebellum of children about the age of 12 years.

Radiography is very important in the diagnosis and localization of these lesions. CT scanning is highly accurate in their detection and has largely replaced studies such as pneumoencephalography, but arteriography still plays a role in demonstrating the vascular supply of tumors shown by CT.

METASTASES. These are common and probably account for about 10% of all intracranial neoplasms. They often are multiple, a useful distinction from the solitary primary neoplasm. Most are blood-borne from such primaries as the lung, breast, kidney, and gastrointestinal tract. Rarely, there is direct spread; e.g., carcinoma of the ethmoids.

ACOUSTIC NEUROMA. This is an uncommon benign tumor with a very slow rate of growth, usually presenting late in life. It arises from the nerve sheath of the eighth cranial nerve. As it grows, it enlarges and destroys the internal auditory meatus; this may be seen on plain films of the area. CT scanning and other organ-imaging methods may be used to demonstrate the tumor itself.

MENINGIOMA. This tumor accounts for about 20% of all intracranial neoplasms and also occurs in the spinal canal. It can arise anywhere where meninges are present; e.g., parasagittal, over brain convexity, sphenoidal ridge. Its highest incidence is in middle-aged adults. Although initially a well-encapsulated benign tumor, it may recur with malignant potential if incompletely removed. Because it may grow slowly, the brain often has time to accommodate, so the tumor may be very large when the patient first presents. It usually is highly vascular and, therefore, may cause changes in the bones of the vault due to the enlarged diploic veins draining from the tumor. CT scanning and angiography will show the lesion. Isotope scanning also is used, as these tumors usually are very "hot."

Trauma

The central nervous system, both brain and spinal cord, are well protected from damage. Not only are they enclosed in an almost complete bony case but this is lined with the tough dura mater. In addition, there is the mechanical buffering effect of the cerebrospinal fluid, and, within the cranial cavity, the falx and tentorium help to prevent undue movement of the brain.

BONE. Sufficient force applied to the skull will cause fractures of various types. Often there is a simple *crack* fracture. A severe localized blow to the vault will cause *depression* of the fragments, with resulting damage to the brain underneath. Sometimes the force is sufficient to cause *penetration* of the vault, allowing air and foreign material to enter the cranial cavity and possibly the brain. Air may also enter the intracranial space through fractures of the cribriform plate or the paranasal sinuses. These latter fractures allow escape of CSF into the nasal cavity (rhinorrhea). The value of radiography in displaying these injuries is obvious.

Bony injury to the vertebral column usually takes the form of compression fractures of the vertebral bodies. If the force is excessive there may be dislocations between the vertebral bodies, often associated with fractures. "Whiplash injury" is a term used to describe trauma to the cervical spine, usually as a result of a car accident in which the head is suddenly propelled forward and then overcorrection occurs in the reverse direction. Often these injuries show little or no change on plain film radiography, but in severe cases there may be compression fractures of the vertebral bodies.

BRAIN. The degree of injury will be related to the severity of the trauma. With a relatively mild blow there will be edema and some localized intracerebral bleeding at the site of injury (contusion). Sometimes the damage to the brain is found opposite the point of impact (contrecoup injury). "Punch-drunk" is a term used to describe chronic extensive brain damage due to multiple minor injuries; e.g., in persons who have boxed for many years. "Concussion" is the clinical state following head injury where there is loss of consciousness and temporary paralysis of the body. Severe damage to the brain will lead to marked loss of consciousness (coma), and if this is severe enough the patient eventually will die.

VESSELS. Vascular damage may result from trauma. Injury to the brain nearly always causes some bleeding from the damaged cortex into the *subarachnoid space*. Of more importance are extradural and subdural hematomas.

An *extradural hematoma* is due to tearing of the meningeal vessels so that bleeding occurs between the bone and the dura. As this bleeding is arterial, the natural history usually is short, a matter of some hours, with a fatal outcome if the condition is not diagnosed and urgently treated by surgery. Even if the condition is recognized early, it still carries a mortality of about 30%. Owing to the rapidity of the deterioration of the patient, radiography often plays little part in the diagnosis except possibly for plain skull films to localize the fracture site.

A *subdural hematoma* is due to a tear of the veins between the dura and arachnoid maters. This bleeding is slow, and often it is some hours or even a day or two before the acute hematoma is large enough to cause compression of the underlying brain. The condition of *chronic* subdural hematoma, due to a very slow bleed, is seen in people who have repeated falls; e.g., alcoholics, the elderly. These chronic hematomas often enlarge due to increased osmosis from the products produced by the breakdown of blood.

Radiography plays an important role in the diagnosis and assessment of head injuries, with the exception of the extradural hematoma. Previously, angiography was of great value but today CT scanning, where available, is the investigation of choice. It can give invaluable information about edema or hemorrhage of the injured brain and show the displacements due to bleeding, either into the subdural space or within the brain itself.

SPINAL CORD. The spinal cord may be damaged or completely divided by severe fracture dislocations of the vertebrae. Direct penetrating injury, e.g., from a bullet, is rare. Injuries to the lower cervical spine result in complete paralysis of all four limbs and of the trunk (quadriplegia). As the nerves to the diaphragm (phrenic) arise from the upper cervical cord, diaphragmatic movement usually is maintained, insuring breathing. More inferior lesions result in various degrees of sensory and motor loss in the lower limbs, together with disturbances of bowel and bladder function (paraplegia).

Infections

Infections can involve either the central nervous system itself or its coverings, the meninges. The infections may be generalized or they may be localized as abscesses.

MENINGITIS. This is inflammation of the meninges, and usually is due to a bacterial cause. The infection is either blood-borne, e.g., meningococcal meningitis, or occurs by direct spread, e.g., from a local osteomyelitis, by a penetrating wound. Inflammation of the meninges can also follow the introduction of a foreign substance into the subarachnoid space; e.g., contrast medium for myelography. This is called a "chemical meningitis" and may result in the formation of adhesions between the meningeal coverings.

ENCEPHALITIS. This is inflammation of the brain. It is not common, and it nearly always is due to a virus; e.g., mumps. "Myelitis" refers to a similar condition of the spinal cord.

ABSCESS. Abscesses may either occur within the brain or be associated with the meninges. A collection of pus between the bone and its underlying dura is called an *epidural* abscess. Sometimes the infection is blood-borne, having embolized from a septic lesion elsewhere in the body. Occasionally, the infection is introduced by a direct route; e.g., from an infected nasal sinus. An untreated brain abscess eventually will rupture into the subarachnoid space or the ventricular system, leading to wide-spread meningitis, nearly always fatal.

Miscellaneous

CEREBRAL ATROPHY (GENERALIZED). This is due to loss of neurons and is seen with increasing frequency in persons over the age of 60 years. It occurs particularly in persons who have widespread arteriosclerosis, which presumably limits the amount of oxygen available to the brain. Affected patients show intellectual impairment; e.g., poor memory, unusual behavior. Occasionally it is seen in younger persons (presenile atrophy). As the brain in cerebral atrophy becomes smaller there is shrinkage of the gyri and some enlargement of the ventricles. These changes can be well demonstrated by CT scanning, so the use of air studies to diagnose this condition now has been largely abandoned.

EPILEPSY (GRAND MAL). This is the condition known as "fits" and its etiology is not known. It is due to excessive uncoordinated discharges from the neurons of the cerebral cortex, leading to loss of consciousness for a short time accompanied by convulsions. At least half of the people affected by epilepsy have some warning (aura) of the onset of an attack. A small group of patients have transient loss of consciousness without convulsions (petit mal). Susceptible persons usually have their first attack of epilepsy before the age of 18 years.

A much smaller group of patients acquire epilepsy. Acquired epilepsy may follow brain damage or it may be the presenting symptom of a cerebral neoplasm. The convulsions often start in a local area of the body, e.g., the hand, before becoming widespread (focal fits). Radiography plays little role in the investigation of epilepsy unless an acquired cause is suspected.

MIGRAINE. This is a condition in which patients suffer from very severe headaches, often accompanied by dislike of light (photophobia) and vomiting. It usually has no organic cause, but occasionally may be associated with cerebral aneurysms or angiomas, so radiography may play a role in excluding these.

MULTIPLE SCLEROSIS. This is a common degenerative disease of the central nervous system of unknown cause. It usually first manifests itself in early adult life, affecting more women than men. The disease involves the brain and spinal cord in a random fashion. It results in local scarring (gliosis) and recurs intermittently. Therefore, these patients present in many different ways and have periods when the disease is stationary, alternating with periods of deterioration. Death is usually due to complicating infection, either pneumonia or of the renal tract. Radiology plays no part in the diagnosis.

PARKINSON'S DISEASE. This is a disorder of the motor system due to degeneration of the basal ganglia, usually associated with senility. Patients show increasing rigidity of movement, associated with persistent uncontrollable shaking of the affected limbs.

SYRINGOMYELIA. This is a rare disease of young adults in which there is degeneration of the gray matter of the spinal cord, usually in the cervical or upper dorsal area. This leads to the formation of a cystic cavity, which enlarges, pressing on the remaining cord tissues. Patients present with loss of sensation and often with neuropathic joints in the upper limbs. Radiography plays a role in demonstrating the enlargement of the cord and the presence of the cystic cavity.

9 / ENDOCRINE SYSTEM

ALTHOUGH there are many diseases of the endocrine glands, only those producing changes visible on x-rays will be described. Some of the lesions are local due to local effects from tumor growth. However, excessive production of a hormone can cause striking widespread changes.

Adrenal Glands

The adrenal glands are best radiographically examined by CT scanning, as they are well demonstrated in their upper abdomen position.

CORTEX. Overactivity of the cortex causes "Cushing's syndrome." Affected patients develop obesity, hypertension, and diabetes. Females show excessive growth of hair (hirsutism). Osteoporosis also develops and this can be shown by radiography. Patients with Cushing's syndrome are prone to infection due to impaired immunity, and radiography may show unsuspected infective lesions; e.g., osteomyelitis. Prolonged steroid therapy produces similar changes.

Underactivity of the cortex is known as "Addison's disease." Affected patients show a clinical picture opposite to Cushing's syndrome. Thus, they lose weight, their blood pressure is low, and often they develop circulatory collapse and die if not treated. The condition is due to destruction or atrophy of the adrenal glands. Previous tuberculous infection used to be the most common cause and x-rays would show calcification in the glands. Today, secondary carcinoma has become a more frequent cause of Addison's disease.

MEDULLA. Two tumors arise in the adrenal medulla. The "pheochromocytoma" is benign and occurs mainly in adults. The "neuroblastoma" is a highly malignant tumor of early childhood.

The pheochromocytoma secretes epinephrine-like substances, intermittently causing episodic hypertension. The blood pressure often reaches very high levels and untreated patients die of vascular complications; e.g., intracerebral hemorrhage. Diagnosis is made on biochemical grounds, and the role of radiography is localization of the tumor. In addition to CT scanning, angiography may be performed, as these tumors usually are highly vascular. Preoperative localization is vitally important, as about 20% of the tumors occur in an ectopic site, usually on the posterior abdominal wall.

The neuroblastoma usually causes considerable enlargement of the adrenal gland. Radiography will show this soft tissue mass, often containing microcalcifications. These tumors metastasize readily, especially to bone, and the prognosis is poor.

Pancreas

DIABETES MELLITUS. This well-known endocrine disease is due to a *lack* of insulin, which leads to disturbance of glucose metabolism. Tissue use and storage of glucose are impaired, so the level of glucose in the blood rises considerably (hyperglycemia). If these patients are not treated, they eventually go into coma and die. Diabetics develop extensive vascular disease, and radiography may play a role in demonstrating the extent of this. Diabetics are also prone to infection, particularly by gas-forming organisms; the gas may be shown by plain films.

ISLET CELL TUMORS. These rare neoplasms produce an *excess* of insulin, which leads to abnormally low levels of blood glucose (hypoglycemia), which may also result in coma and death. Angiography may play a role in the localization of these tumors.

ZOLLINGER-ELLISON SYNDROME. This syndrome already has been referred to as a cause of peptic ulceration. It is due to another type of islet cell tumor that excretes excessive amounts of the hormone gastrin, stimulating the gastric cells to produce large volumes of gastric juice. Radiography occasionally is useful in localizing the tumor before surgery.

Parathyroid Gland

Overactivity of the parathyroids is known as "hyperparathyroidism." Owing to excessive output of the hormone parathormone, the osteoclasts are overstimulated, resulting in destruction of the skeleton, leading to an increase in the level of the serum calcium. This excess serum calcium leads to increased renal excretion, which predisposes to stone formation, so the patients may present with renal colic. Affected patients may also complain of bone pain and nonspecific symptoms; e.g., vomiting.

The lesions of hyperparathyroidism can be demonstrated radiographically, especially if the condition is advanced. There may be osteoporosis and consequent pathologic fracturing of bones. Films of the fingers are particularly useful in detecting early subperiosteal bone absorption. Sometimes there are cystic areas in the bone (osteoclastomas). Radiography of the renal tract may show calcified stones and their complications; e.g., obstruction. Sometimes the excess serum calcium leads to deposition of calcification in unusual areas, "metastatic" or "dystrophic" calcification, which is readily demonstrated on plain films.

Radiography can make the initial diagnosis of this condition by showing the widespread skeletal changes. Occasionally it is used to locate the parathyroid tumor prior to surgery. This often is difficult, as the tumors usually are small. Although most of them are found in the parathyroids, the occasional aberrant tumor in the mediastinum can cause diagnostic problems.

"Secondary hyperparathyroidism" is a condition seen in patients with chronic renal disease. Due to the disturbance of calcium and phosphate metabolism in these patients there is excessive output of parathormone, which leads to a condition similar to that seen with a primary tumor.

Pituitary Gland

BENIGN ADENOMA (CHROMOPHOBE). Many neoplasms of the pituitary gland do not secrete excess hormone and so do not give rise to generalized or distant changes, but they may produce local changes because of their size. A large pituitary adenoma will press on the floor of the pituitary fossa, causing ballooning and destruction, with erosion of the posterior clinoid processes. Because the optic chiasma lies immediately anterior to the pituitary stalk, many of these patients present with visual disturbances in addition to symptoms of raised intracranial pressure.

EOSINOPHILIC ADENOMA. These benign adenomas secrete growth hormone. The size of the adenoma and its hormonal activity do not correlate, so a normal-sized pituitary may have an active eosinophilic adenoma within it. If the excess growth hormone is secreted *before* fusion of the epiphyses, the patient continues to grow, especially in height, giving rise to "gigantism." Excess secretion of growth hormone *after* fusion of the epiphyses causes hypertrophy of the soft tissues, so these patients show changes such as big hands and feet, an enlarged heart, thickening of the heel pad, and greatly enlarged frontal sinuses. Because of the cartilage on the mandibular head there is further growth in the mandible at this site, so the mandible projects forward. If the adenoma is large, it will cause local changes in the pituitary fossa. Many of the general and local features of acromegaly can be demonstrated by radiography.

DIABETES INSIPIDUS. Patients with this condition pass large volumes of urine because of a lack of antidiuretic hormone. This is due to destruction of the posterior pituitary gland by a variety of causes, secondary carcinoma being the most common. Diabetes insipidus may also occur as a complication of "Hand-Schüller-Christian syndrome."

Thyroid Gland

The thyroid cannot be visualized on plain film radiography, although sometimes areas of calcification may be seen within it. If the gland enlarges, it may press on the trachea, causing displacement or narrowing. Occasionally, the thyroid enlarges by extending into the superior mediastinum. Isotope scanning is the most useful diagnostic organ-imaging method.

GOITER. "Goiter" means thyroid gland enlargement without specifying its cause. Many goiters are due to lack of iodine in the diet. Such goiters contain large amounts of colloid and often undergo partial calcification.

OVERACTIVITY. The condition of "thyrotoxicosis" (Graves' disease) is due to excessive production of thyroxine. There rarely are any radiographic changes. However, radiographers should be aware that patients with thyrotoxicosis often are unduly agitated and nervous, an effect of the excessive output of thyroxine.

UNDERACTIVITY. If there is a deficiency of thyroxine in infancy, the condition of "cretinism" develops. The child fails to develop both physically and mentally. Of importance to the radiographer is the gross disturbance of skeletal development so that the epiphyses appear late and have an abnormal structure.

Thyroxine deficiency later in life leads to the condition of "myxedema." Affected patients are lethargic.

CARCINOMA. Carcinoma of the thyroid is a rare condition. Its metastases may be widespread, e.g., lungs and skeleton, and radiography can detect them.

10 / BLOOD AND RETICULOENDOTHELIAL SYSTEM

A WIDE RANGE OF LESIONS affect these systems, and most are of little or no significance to radiographers. Malignancies are the diseases most likely to be encountered. These often are generalized and multicentric in origin.

Anemia

When the amount of hemoglobin in the blood is lowered, the patient is said to have anemia. This is due to many causes, e.g., poor diet, and those of importance to the radiographer are the following.

CHRONIC BLOOD LOSS. There is continuous slow loss of blood, nearly always from the gastrointestinal tract; e.g., peptic ulcer, carcinoma. Patients with anemia due to chronic blood loss often have contrast examinations to detect the source of bleeding.

PERNICIOUS ANEMIA. Due to gastric mucosal atrophy, patients with this anemia fail to secrete hydrochloric acid and intrinsic factor (achlorhydria), which prevents absorption of vitamin B_{12}, essential for red cell maturation. The incidence of gastric carcinoma is greatly increased in these patients.

HEMOLYTIC ANEMIA. Due to defects in either the red blood cell or its hemoglobin there is an increased rate of destruction of these cells. Examples are "sickle cell" anemia occurring in blacks and "thalassemia" occurring in populations around the Mediterranean Sea. Due to increased demands, the bone marrow hypertrophies, so skeletal changes develop. Sickle cell anemia is also associated with infarction of various organs. Radiography, therefore, plays a role in demonstrating the complications of these anemias.

Leukemias

These are malignancies of the white blood cells, which may be either acute or chronic. As different types of white cells may undergo neoplastic change, the various leukemias are named after the predominant cell; e.g., lymphatic, myelocytic. There is great multiplication of the abnormal cells in the bone marrow, which is reflected in greatly increased numbers of them in the circulating blood. Due to the space occupied in the marrow by these neoplastic cells, the production of the other corpuscles, red blood cells and platelets, is decreased. These patients, therefore, are anemic, their blood fails to clot properly, and they are prone to infections because of lack of normal cells to fight bacteria. Later, other organs are invaded by the malignant cells.

The main incidence of leukemia is in early childhood and again in the elderly. Its etiology usually is not known. Exposure to excessive irradiation can cause leukemia, but most patients have no such history. As with other malignant neoplasms, the untreated patient eventually will die of the condition. The course of the disease varies markedly according to the type. Thus, some patients die in weeks whereas others, e.g., those with chronic lymphatic leukemia, may survive for years.

Radiologic changes are restricted mainly to the skeleton. As the leukemic cells invade the bones, they cause destructive lesions. In growing children there may be a thin radiolucent line beneath the metaphyses, due to infiltration by the abnormal cells. Infiltration of other organs, e.g., spleen, may enlarge them. There may be nonspecific changes; e.g., pneumonia due to diminished resistance to infection.

Myelomatosis (Myeloma)

This is a malignant neoplasm of the plasma cells in the bone marrow with a poor prognosis, most patients dying in less than five years. It is uncommon, although there is evidence to suggest that its incidence is increasing. It rarely is seen in patients under the age of 50 years. About half the patients have an unusual protein in their urine (Bence Jones protein), which redissolves on boiling, unlike other proteins that precipitate; e.g., egg white. Myeloma usually remains localized to the skeleton, and radiography will show evidence of bone destruction with osteoporosis. Classically, the areas of bone destruction have a punched-out appearance with clear-cut margins, unlike the more-ill-defined edges of metastases. As the bone destruction continues there is an increasing number of pathologic fractures. A significant number of these patients develop paraplegia due to overgrowth of the marrow in the vertebral column pressing on the spinal cord.

Lymphomas

These are malignant neoplasms of the lymph nodes and associated tissues; e.g., spleen. There are several different types, the best known being *Hodgkin's disease. Lymphosarcoma* is another variety. These tumors usually start in one group of lymph nodes, enlarging them. Histology reveals that the normal architecture of the lymph nodes is replaced with abnormal cells. The condition then spreads or arises separately in other groups of lymph nodes, and the spleen eventually is involved in at least 75% of cases. The patients usually present with a mass of locally enlarged nodes but soon exhibit general symptoms; e.g., malaise, raised temperature. The disease almost always is fatal, although the prognosis in any individual case depends on the type of lymphoma, some patients surviving for many years.

The principal role of radiography is to demonstrate the extent of the disease (staging). This is important, as the staging greatly influences treatment.

Thus, plain films of the chest are taken, searching for hilar node involvement. CT scanning of both the mediastinum and the abdomen is used to detect enlarged nodes in those areas. Lower limb lymphangiography often is performed to demonstrate the involvement of the iliac and para-aortic nodes. Plain films will show if the disease has spread to the skeleton.

Metastases

Metastatic carcinoma is far more common as a cause of lymph node enlargement than any of the primary diseases. The nodes usually involved, especially in the early stages, are the regional ones draining the organ containing the primary. Due to the course of the thoracic duct, nodes in the lower left neck may be enlarged by metastases from intra-abdominal carcinomas.

Storage Diseases

This is a group of rare diseases in which metabolic defects lead to the storage of abnormal substances, especially in the reticuloendothelial system and bone marrow. Plain films may show gross enlargement of the liver and spleen, and bones may be widened and weakened. In some of these lesions there is local bony destruction by the stored materials; e.g., histiocytosis X (Hand-Schüller-Christian disease). If the latter involves the base of the skull, it causes diabetes insipidus.

Thymomas

These are rare tumors of the thymus usually occurring in adults. Most are benign and often are found by chance on a plain chest x-ray taken for another reason. About a quarter of them are associated with skeletal muscle weakness (myasthenia gravis).

INDEX